The Journey

A Journal of God's Trustworthiness Through a Cancer Journey

by Lee Ann Martin

OUTCOME PUBLISHING

The Journey
by Lee Ann Martin

Published by Outcome Publishing
6433 Blue Grosbeak Circle
Bradenton, Florida 34202
www.gooutcome.com

First Edition

Printed in the United States of America

Dedication

This book is dedicated to the hundreds of friends and family from all across the world that prayed for us and encouraged us through this difficult journey.

You will never know how much your encouragement means to us.

Introduction

When Keith went into the hospital in July, 2009, our church was overwhelmed with people calling and trying to get information on him. They asked if I would consider doing a page on the church's website to do updates so people would have a central place to go to get information.

What started as an information tool turned into a great network of prayer warriors that literally carried us through the next 24 months of chemotherapy, surgery, and more chemotherapy. The first week that it was up, the page had over 3000 hits.

I have put this together in book form for the sole purpose of my children and grandchildren having a written record of the events of this journey, and the evidence of God's faithfulness through it.

You might find typos and bad grammar, which I apologize for in advance. I am not an author, just a wife who told a story through a journal about an incredible journey of faith.

Before we begin, this is a synopsis of the story:

Keith began having severe pain in his back in March, 2009. We went to several doctors, he had cortisone injections, and the pain would get better, and then come back with a vengeance. In mid-July, we were with a group on our Navajo mission trip and the pain became completely unmanageable for Keith. We made the decision to fly him home. Keith came home and went to the doctor for more tests. They finally ran a CT scan and discovered that Keith had a large mass in his abdomen. They immediately admitted him to the hospital in order to monitor him and help with the pain. He was admitted to the hospital on Friday, July 17, 2009.

The doctors at the time were pretty sure that it was lymphoma. The tumor was quite large - 4" x 6", which is why it caused so much pain. They did a biopsy to determine what kind of cancer it was. The test results were inconclusive, so the sample was sent to the Mayo Clinic for evaluation. The results from Mayo showed that it was a Seminoma, a form of testicular cancer. None of the doctors had suspected it because of Keith's age (okay, he's not OLD, but they usually see this in younger men.) The good news is that it is very treatable and has a very high cure rate (95%)

We did the whole testicular cancer thing in reverse, so then they did an ultrasound and discovered that his right testicle was completely full of tumors. The first of August he had the diseased testicle removed. That is not a surgery that he would recommend to anyone!

He went through 4 rounds of chemotherapy in August-November. After that he was referred to Moffitt Cancer Center in Tampa, and the decision was made to do surgery to remove the remainder of the tumor. This was a very difficult, very long surgery called Retroperitoneal Lymph Node Dissection. It was done on March 18, and Keith was in surgery over 9 hours!

The pathology report from the surgery showed that the tumor still had cancer cells remaining, so he began 3 more rounds of chemotherapy in April. That led to those glorious words: “No Cancer Evident” in August.

On Sunday afternoon, July 19, 2009, at 3:15 in the afternoon, I had a very personal, but very profound experience. It was 2 days after they had found the mass in Keith’s abdomen. I was sitting in the hospital room with him as he slept. I was absolutely scared to death as to what we might be facing, and was praying and seeking God for direction and peace. At 3:15, (I know the time, because the event was so profound that I checked it. The image of that clock is branded on my brain.) I felt the Lord saying to me, "He's going to come through this, but it is going to be a very difficult journey." I never shared that because it was so personal and not something that I knew many people could understand. However, it was those few moments that brought me peace through those very difficult months.

At the first printing of this book, we thought the cancer journey was behind us. But, as this book went to press in early November, we found out that the cancer had returned. Through an amazing series of events we ended up with Dr. Lawrence Einhorn at the University of Indiana Medical Center. We spent two very long, cold months in Indianapolis for Keith to have a stem cell transplant, and once again it was proclaimed that Keith was cancer free.

God had another plan, however, as in March of 2011 we found out that the cancer had returned.

Then, on July 15, 2011, Keith was ushered into Heaven. He was a victim of what should have been a cureable cancer...one of only 300 deaths from testicular cancer this year.

So, while the journey turned out differently than we had first thought, it was important to me to finish this book, and finish the story. I have also included entries from my private journal that I did not put on the blog.

It was also very important to Keith to give testicular cancer patients a place to come to find out information about treatments and their effects. It is my hope that this book will provide that.

I hope you enjoy our journey.

The Journey

Monday, July 20

The church has asked me to provide a page on the web site to provide a daily update on Keith.

In case there are some who are not aware of what we are dealing with, Keith has had severe pain in his back for a couple of months. We have been to several doctors, he has had cortisone injections, and the pain would get better, and then come back with a vengeance. This past week, we were with a group on our Navajo mission trip and the pain became completely unmanageable for Keith. We made the decision to fly him home, and I chose to stay with the group to lead the remainder of the tour. Keith came home and went to the doctor for more tests. They finally ran a CT scan on Friday and have discovered that Keith has a large mass in his abdomen. They immediately admitted him to the hospital in order to monitor him and help with the pain. He has been resting now, and claims "Uncle Morphine" is his new best friend!

The doctors are pretty sure that this is lymphoma. The tumor is quite large - 4" x 6", which is why it caused so much pain. They did a biopsy this morning to determine what kind of cancer it is, then based on that they will determine the course of treatment. We will not have the results back until as late as Wednesday.

We are doing okay. The realization of what we are dealing with has hit us at different times. The biopsy was a difficult experience for Keith today (he was awake during it and could hear all that was going on). I'm still a little numb, but am acutely aware that the one I love most on this earth has cancer. I can honestly say that a week ago that word wasn't even a part of my vocabulary!

Josh is coming home tomorrow. He already had a trip scheduled, so looks like God has been working in the background preparing the way for all of this! Bethany will be coming in the first of August.

Today's prayer requests:

1. Wisdom for the doctors as they are analyzing the tissue
2. Wisdom for us as to the treatment plan and where we need to be. There are many great cancer centers around...I just want to be sure we are at the best.
3. All of us as the reality of cancer slowly sinks in.

Tuesday, July 21

Not much news to report today. Keith is comfortable. They are weaning him off of the Morphine in order to get him to the place where he can be discharged when the time comes. Don't worry, they are replacing the morphine with other, super duper pain meds. His one plea is that he does not have to go back to the pain!

The Oncologist today said that he hoped to have the results by tomorrow morning. If they do, and can confirm a course of treatment, it is my understanding that they will begin the first treatment in the hospital. No one will commit, until they really know what this monster is, but sometimes they will guess (when I push them a little!!) The only hold up would be if this is something that can not be identified here, then it will have to be sent off, which will take longer.

They have some other tests that they will need to run as routine, to be sure there are not cancer cells anywhere else. They don't suspect that there are, because his blood work looks great, but they have to be sure.

We have had a little mix-up regarding the Oncologist that was supposed to be treating Keith. We are working with our PCP to get that straightened out. Just one more headache I wish that we didn't have!

Today's prayer requests:

1. Still pray about the analyzing of the tissue - quick, but accurate analysis!
2. That we will end up with the absolute best Oncologist for Keith and his situation.
3. That they will find the right pain "cocktail" so that he can come home when the time is right.
4. When the new tests are done, that they will find no new cancer cells.
5. Complete healing. We are not asking God to take away this journey we know we need to travel, but to bring us through to the other side so Keith can quickly go back to doing what he loves - leading people to worship God.

Thanks for all the emails and calls. Keith really enjoys reading the emails on his "blueberry." Your words and prayers are very encouraging.

Hopefully tomorrow we will have a little more direction!!

Wednesday, July 22

I know many of you are going to be checking this page today to see about Keith's diagnosis, so I wanted to go ahead and write early. I have good news and bad news. The bad news is that we still don't have a diagnosis. The pathology report basically came back that it is cancer (I should be a Pathologist...I think I could have given that info!) They have had to send it off in order to identify exactly what it is. The doctor says that this is not uncommon. It will potentially be Friday or next Tuesday before we know for sure. What does this mean? Well, our kids were praying that they would find that this was a big cyst of some kind. Looks like that's not the case. However, this does NOT mean that he has some kind of exotic, rare cancer (it doesn't mean that he doesn't, but...well you know.) All it means is that the findings were inconclusive. The doctor still thinks we are dealing with lymphoma, and to be honest, that's our best scenario.

The good news...we have found an Oncologist that we really like and we think has a good plan. The way this all happened I believe is a direct result of all of your prayers. This man came highly recommended to us, and came in last night at 8:15 and stayed until 9:45 to meet with us and walk us through everything. We got more information from him in that time than we have received since we arrived at the hospital on Friday. And for those of you that were concerned...he said that at any point that he feels that this is something beyond the scope of his practice, he will send us to Moffitt or MDAnderson. That's getting the cart before the horse, but it made me feel better. I felt such peace in talking to him, and it was like a huge weight had been lifted off of me that this decision had been made.

The doctors think Keith might be able to come home tomorrow. That would be great, as long as all has been accomplished that needs to be. He will probably get the chemo port today. Wow, I really can't believe that "chemo port" is now a part of my vocabulary (sorry, the realization still comes in waves.)

Josh got in yesterday. It is great to have him here.

Today's prayer requests are the same as yesterday, pretty much, but with one of them answered!! From here on out, I may just add to the list each day.

Today's prayer requests:

1. Still pray about the analyzing of the tissue - quick, but accurate analysis! Our prayer is still that we are dealing with lymphoma.
2. That we will end up with the absolute best Oncologist for Keith and his situation. ANSWERED!!
3. That they will find the right pain "cocktail" so that he can come home when the time is right.
4. When the new tests are done, that they will find no new cancer cells.
5. Complete healing. We are not asking God to take away this journey we know we need to travel, but to bring us through to the other side so Keith can quickly go back to doing what he loves - leading people to worship God.

I'm on my way to the hospital now, so if there is any more news this afternoon, I will update.

I cannot thank you enough that you guys are there and praying for us. The first day this page was up, it had 655 hits. You are absolutely strength for us during this difficult time.

Thursday, July 23

Keith is home! I look at him in there, sitting in his chair, playing with the dog, and it sure seems like things are back to normal. I know they are far from normal, but I am giving myself this moment!

Still no diagnosis, but this afternoon we go for a PET Scan. A quick prayer request for those of you that are reading this before 3 pm ET - we need his blood sugar to be below 200 in order for them to give him the test. The blood sugar is elevated as they have already started him on some steroids to try and shrink the tumor or at least stunt its growth!

Tomorrow is our first official visit with the Oncologist. If we have any news as far as a diagnosis, I will let you know as soon as I know. It may be as late as next week before we get the final word. They have scheduled to have the chemo port put in on Monday so that we will be sitting on ready when we know what this beast is!

Today's prayer requests:

1. Still pray about the analyzing of the tissue - quick, but accurate analysis! Our prayer is still that we are dealing with lymphoma.
2. That we will end up with the absolute best Oncologist for Keith and his situation. ANSWERED!!
3. That they will find the right pain "cocktail" so that he can come home when the time is right. ANSWERED!!
4. When the new tests are done, that they will find no new cancer cells.
5. Complete healing. We are not asking God to take away this journey we know we need to travel, but to bring us through to the other side so Keith can quickly go back to doing what he loves - leading people to worship God.
6. I'm a little nervous about the "pain management" from home. Please pray that I can keep it all straight and him pain free!

Friday, July 24

Well, we are one week into this journey, and it seems like we have been traveling it for about a year! One week ago today, I was standing on a street corner in Gallup, NM (where we had been on a mission trip), listening to the doctor tell me on the phone that he was pretty sure that my husband had cancer. I thought he had a kidney stone! Turns out he was right, but we still don't know what kind!

Okay, so now I am frustrated. We were told this morning that the test results would be in as late as the end of next week. With apologies to those in the health community (in case I tell this wrong), it is my understanding that because they couldn't remove an entire node, it is difficult to determine the architecture of the cell, so even the most simple of diagnosis oftentimes has to be sent away for analysis. Now I'm in a quandary as to whether to sit quietly and wait, or to raise a little stink to try and get the diagnosis. It was a rhetorical question, actually, as I know I just need to wait (but maybe not quietly!!) These doctors and pathologists don't seem to realize that they have in their possession the most important test results in the world!!

Last night was a rough night. His pain broke through at about 3 am, so I called the doctor (so thankful for a kind and patient PCP) and he had me increase the pain meds. I think we have the formula figured out now, although he is a little loopy for awhile right after he takes it.

Bethany comes in tonight. So both our kids will be here for the weekend. I think we are going to cloister away and just have some fun watching movies, playing games and just being together. I probably won't update until Monday (chemo port at 7 am). In the meantime, please move the diagnosis to the top of the prayer list, but most importantly that it be accurate!

We love you all. Since Monday, Keith and I combined have received over 500 emails. Please don't stop! All of your notes and prayers of encouragement really make his day. Just please understand if we don't reply. I know you do.

Hopefully this time next week we will know a little more.

Monday, July 27

So, here we are in the second week of the Keith Martin journey. The week end was great - so good to have Josh and Bethany both home. We played games, went to a movie, and just had fun being together. Friday night we had a precious prayer time together. Bethany went back to Auburn yesterday, and Josh heads back to Dallas tomorrow.

This morning they put the chemo port in. Just a little bump next to his collarbone. I guess I expected something a little more menacing. He can finally shower without having to wrap his arm in cellophane (pic line), so he is very glad about that. The anesthesia really socked him...Josh and I took him to get something for breakfast and he kept falling asleep. The best one was when he was drinking his hot tea and before he could set the cup down, he fell asleep. I grabbed the cup and made the decision to get him home for a nap!

His spirits are good. He is still picking on us and playing practical jokes. Typical Keith stuff.

Tomorrow we have to have a heart scan (muga scan, I think it's called), just to be sure his heart is okay to withstand the chemo. They are definitely getting all the pieces in place to jump on this monster once they get a diagnosis. Still thinking that will happen by Friday. He had the PET scan on Thursday, and it should be read today.

Thanks for your prayers for me. I'm a little calmer today about waiting on the diagnosis. Every doctor we have encountered says that this is not uncommon, so I guess I will have to take a breath, sit back and wait! We still have a slight hope that it might come in tomorrow. At this point the Oncologist is planning starting treatment on Monday, August 3.

Today's prayer requests:

1. Still pray about the analyzing of the tissue - quick, but accurate analysis! Our prayer is still that we are dealing with lymphoma or something that can be treated easily.
2. When the new tests are done, that they will find no new cancer cells.
3. Complete healing. We are not asking God to take away this journey we know we need to travel, but to bring us through to the other side so Keith can quickly go back to doing what he loves - leading people to worship God.

Tuesday, July 28

Sorry I am so late updating this today, but I have just returned from Tampa taking Josh to the airport. Keith had the Muga scan today, checking the functionality of his heart. I think they did this because one of his veins is collapsed from the tumor and they want to be sure the surrounding veins can carry the load.

So, we have chemo port in place, and all of the tests complete. Now we just need the diagnosis. We did get a bit of news today, in that the PET scan seems to support the lymphoma diagnosis. We just need to know which lymphoma in order to know the treatment protocol.

Funny on Keith: The doctor has given him an Ambien prescription in case he needs it to sleep. Last night he was having trouble sleeping and took one of those pills around 3:30 am. We got up around 8 am, and he was SO goofy! He didn't know what day it was, couldn't stay focused, mumbled - I was really worried! Then I talked with the doctor who said it is imperative that he get at least 8 hours of sleep when he takes that. Sure enough, right after lunch he was back to his old self, and would not believe that he had done anything strange!

The Lord is using each of you in our lives during this time. I can never thank you enough for all of the prayers, verses, and encouragement that you have sent us. One of the neatest things for me are when people quote Keith's words back to him that he said to them during difficult times. God is sustaining us, and I feel we are truly being lifted on your prayers.

Today's prayer requests:

1. Still pray about the analyzing of the tissue - quick, but accurate analysis! Our prayer is still that we are dealing with lymphoma or something that can be treated easily.
2. When the new tests are done, that they will find no new cancer cells.
3. I tend to worry about the amount of pain medication that he is taking. I know that can cause problems down the road. Please pray that God will protect him from any additional complications from it.
4. Complete healing. We are not asking God to take away this journey we know we need to travel, but to bring us through to the other side so Keith can quickly go back to doing what he loves - leading people to worship God.

Wednesday, July 29

Well, we received a little bit of news today. The Radiologist called this morning to let me know that he had been in contact with the Pathologist that had Keith's biopsy. Come to find out, the tests are being done at Mayo Clinic. That made me feel better as far as the facility, but sure do wish they would hurry up! He said the Pathologist said they were still in the process of staining and testing. He did say, however, that the sample is good, so they are not going to have to go back in and do the biopsy again. That's great news, because if we had to do that we'd be in for another 2 week wait! He really feels like we will have the results in a day or so, and is calling them again to be sure they have them as soon as possible.

Another bit of news: he said that the PET scan showed a "hot spot" by Keith's left collarbone. From what I understand, the PET shows the early development of cancer cells. This is what helped to support the Lymphoma suspicion. Our Oncologist has never been able to understand how he could have a mass the size of this one and it not be elsewhere in the body. According to the Radiologist, the Lymphoma diagnosis is better than a Carcinoma. But, we will deal with whatever it is...if we could find out what it is!!

I have enjoyed all of your emails sharing your Ambien stories. Apparently Keith's story is mild compared to what some of you have experienced!

Please continue to pray about the diagnosis. Ask God to really keep that Mayo Pathologist focused and enthralled by Keith's samples!!

Thursday, July 30

Today has been a quiet one. No news from the health front. Keith had the hiccups again last night, and they kept him up a good portion of the night. Today they have not been a problem though.

Our doctor's appointment is at 9:30 am tomorrow morning. We are still praying that we will have a diagnosis by then. I promise that whatever we find out I will post here as soon as we get home. Whatever this is, I want all of you praying about it as soon as possible!!

The quiet day has been nice. I have realized that once Keith starts treatment our lives will change dramatically; at least for the first few weeks (The doctor has already told us he will be a pretty sick boy for the first 2 weeks). So, I figure we have about 3 days left before that dramatic change, so we are enjoying them.

Again, our prayer request is that the diagnosis is available tomorrow, and for strength for us as we face whatever this is.

Friday, July 31

We have a diagnosis! This morning the doctor came in and said, "Well, we have very good news. We have the diagnosis, and it's not what any of us thought!" It seems that the results from Mayo show that this is a Seminoma, a form of testicular cancer. None of the doctors a suspected it because of Keith's age (okay, he's not OLD, but they usually see this in younger men.) The good news is that it is very treatable and has a very high cure rate (95%). The doctor said that Keith would go through the treatment and then move forward and live his life!
The cancer has still not been staged, as we had to do 2 more tests today. The first was a little scary, in that they wanted an MRI of his brain to be sure the cancer had not spread. No reason to suspect that it had, but that would make a difference in the treatment if it had. The second is an ultrasound to be sure there are no additional masses. The only funny in this is that he has to go to a Women's Ultrasound Center for the test...Keith and all the pregnant women!

If the doctor can get all of these results back by Monday afternoon, then Keith will start chemotherapy on Tuesday. The doctor said the treatment would be rough due to the drugs that they have to use, but he again emphasized that given the choice of this or lymphoma, he would definitely take Seminoma, due to the high success with treatment. If there are no complications or further spreading, he feels like the treatment will last around 4 months.

There are lymph nodes in the groin and one by his collarbone that are affected, but the doctor feels like the chemo will take care of all of it. With a cancer mass this size, he did say that it may only shrink to a certain size, and then will have to be surgically removed. If that's the case, he wants us to have that surgery done at Moffitt in Tampa.

When we got in the car after the doctor's appt., Keith looks at me and says..."So...I have MAN cancer." (deep bass voice on the word "man.") This is the same cancer that Lance Armstong had, so Keith thinks he's in good company.

This is obviously still very serious, and we still have a long road to travel, but how thankful we are that it is something that they anticipate will respond well to the treatment and that he can come through and live a normal life. He is just walking around the house saying, "Thank you, Jesus!"

Please pray that the tests today will not show any spread of the cancer, and that all the results will be in so that he can start the treatment on Tuesday. The first round of chemo for this is a 3 day treatment, so if he doesn't get to start on Tuesday, then he will have to wait until the following Monday.

We absolutely give God the glory for these results. I guess the most significant thing, though, is that we were prepared to give him the glory whatever the results. The peace that we have had, largely because of all of your prayers has been amazing. But God, in his graciousness, heard our plea and we are so thankful.

Long entry today. I'll let you know on Monday what the test results are and how we are moving forward. We love you all.

Monday, August 3

Sorry I am so late posting this today, but it is 6 pm, and we have just returned home from our 4 pm doctor's appointment! AND the doctor wasn't running late! He took over an hour and a half to go through everything with us, all the treatment, side effects, scary stuff and positive stuff. I'll try and relay enough that you will know how to pray, but not be overwhelmed with information!

First, the brain scan showed that he does have a brain, and there is no cancer in it. That was a huge relief. The ultrasound did show some testicular tumors, and while that is not great news, it absolutely leaves no question about the Mayo diagnosis. There were also some elevated protein thingys, all of which confirm the diagnosis. So, for all of you medical types out there, it seems Keith has a pure Seminoma. They don't stage these by normal cancer staging, but his is the intermediate level, which means he has a mass larger than 8 cm outside the testicle.

The doctor still feels like this will respond very well to the treatment, but the treatment will be pretty brutal. He won't start the chemotherapy until next Monday, August 10, as each cycle of therapy is 5 days long. He will go for 5 days (5 hours per day). Then he will take two weeks off, where he will still have to go in 3 days a week to get shots to boost his immune system and his blood count. Those 3 weeks is a cycle, and the doctor feels like he will have 3-4 cycles. Then they will do the PET scan and CT scan again to see if the tumor has been obliterated, which is obviously the goal. The doctor is still saying that the cure rate for this is very high, for which we are so thankful.

Today has been a little tough, because while we are still absolutely thankful for the treatable cancer, the reality of the next few months really came into focus today. It's gonna be a tough ride. The doctor went into great detail as to the side effects and potential side effects that Keith will experience.

Keith has already been planning his chemo week, and previewing music is on the top of the list! All of you metro guys, he may have a "Songs from Chemo" list that he can recommend after this is over!

Please pray for the treatment process. I know many of you that are reading this have experienced cancer treatments and can empathize in a way the rest of us can not. We have asked God to do a great work through this, not just in Keith's body, but in the life of our church and in the many friends who have supported us so incredibly. We love you all, and are so thankful for you.

Tuesday, August 4

We had a wonderful, sweet, inspiring prayer time tonight with our church, our deacons, and our staff. The original plan for the prayer time was for the deacons to anoint and pray for Keith. This past weekend Tim offered the invitation for anyone who would like prayer to come and be prayed for. The stories of those that came were inspiring and heart-breaking, but their faith and trust in God was so evident. As we gathered around each of them, with our hands touching them, we brought their needs to the Father's throne.

So, tomorrow I will tell you more about Keith, but tonight I would like to ask this mighty army of prayer warriors to pray for the following, whose stories we heard tonight:

1. James - a young father battling colon and liver cancer
2. Carol - a sweet friend battling colon cancer
3. Cam - a dear woman with a chronic lung infection
4. Ashley - a young mother with cancer recurrence
5. Jackie - a precious staff wife fighting cancer in her hip, lung and brain
6. Mike - a young father with chronic pain in his leg

Keith is scheduled for surgery on Thursday. I'll update you on that tomorrow. Thank you for praying for these friends.

Wednesday, August 5

Today is rather quiet, Keith is trying to get things done and in order before his surgery tomorrow. Part of the treatment for the testicular cancer is the removal of the cancerous testicle. This will be done tomorrow at 2 pm. It is an outpatient surgery, but still requires full anesthesia (and Keith wants as MUCH anesthesia as they will give him!) We should be home by around 5 pm, so I will update on him when we get back.

He will recuperate over the weekend and then begin the chemo on Monday. Definitely going to be a tough week, but when I read back over these entries from the past 2 weeks, I am so glad that we are finally moving forward attacking this thing!

Please pray for the surgery, that it will go as easily as possible, and that his recovery from this will be quick, so he will be ready for the chemo on Monday. Also, please pray for ease in the pain. He's having pain in his back at night again, and we really feel like the tumor is getting larger.

We are already seeing God's hand in the midst of all of this. Thank you so much for your continued prayer support.

Thursday, August 6

Boy, what a day! Keith's spirits were good this morning. We prayed together, then he looked at me and said, "Well, we're breaking up the team today!" You gotta love his sense of humor!

But things were rough from there. The surgery went well, but they did not manage the "tumor pain" while he was there, so by the time we got home he was in blood curdling pain in his back. Forget the pain from just having had a testicle removed, the cancer pain was literally devastating. And the worst part was that I couldn't get any doctors on the phone to tell me how much medicine he could have. The urologist (who is not very high on my list right now) gave him a prescription for Percoset, which doesn't even touch Keith's pain. He knew that Keith was on morphine, but.....okay, I'll stop complaining. ANYWAY we have finally taken the edge off of the back pain tonight, and he has begun to realize that something traumatic has also happened to another part of his body.

All of that to say, I am anticipating a very rough night tonight, so please pray for him. He is really in bad shape, but needs to get some rest. We need all of you tonight. Please pray for pain relief.

Friday, August 7

Thank you so much for all of your kind emails and your prayer support during our difficult time last night. The tumor pain was finally beginning to be managed around 3 am. Then, the attention turned to the incision pain. That, too, is finally managed today, although he is NOT moving from his chair!! His goal is to stand up and walk around 4 pm...we'll see how that goes!

Seeing how awful the pain was from that tumor yesterday just reminded me again of the size of this monster that is inside of him. While yesterday was very difficult, it is good to be moving forward. Yesterday the first piece of this awful disease was removed from his body, and Monday we're going to begin zapping the rest of it!

I guess he is doing better, as right now he is meeting in our Living Room with his Ministry Assistant and Choir President planning the Fall Kick Off Banquet! He's also planning to choose fall choir music and Christmas music during chemo next week! We'll see how it all plays out, but it's nice to see him doing what he loves.

I can't thank you enough for your prayer support last night. Please begin now to pray about next week and the chemo treatment. I don't know what to expect, but you are all a part of our lives now, so I promise to give a full report when we get home on Monday!

Monday, August 10

We have just returned from the first day of chemo, and I am happy to report....it was uneventful!! We met with the nurse this morning and she went over all that would be happening to him the next few weeks, then, we went into the "chemo room," where they put him in a big blue recliner and hooked him up! He pulled out his music and earphones, and previewed music for 5 hours! Aside from a little bit of burning as the chemical went in, he did fine today. They gave him nausea medicine with it, and they told him that he might experience some nausea tonight, but we are armed with 2 different medicines just in case. For those of you from Bradenton, we stopped on the way home at Sweet Berries for a Peach and Banana Concrete...the perfect post chemo treat!

Of course, they had to go over the potential side effects from all of this, everything ranging from lung disease to neuropathy to hearing problems. Some are pretty scary things, but I know that God has carried us to this point, and is still working His plan. My eyes have been opened to the magnitude of this cancer thing, and how many people it affects. Each chair in that room held a different story, most of them overwhelming.

I do have a bit of a funny story from the weekend. You may remember that we had a terrible Thursday night. Well, the doctor had told me that I could give Keith an additional Fentynol patch (50mcg) along with the 100 mcg if needed. Of course, with all the craziness I was trying to give him anything that would help, so I put both patches on him. Well, about midafternoon on Friday, he REALLY turned into a zombie. I mean, scary stuff. He was saying things that didn't make sense, couldn't remember basic things, and I was really getting worried. He was still taking the morphine on a regular basis, same as usual, so I couldn't think of anything that would cause him to be so zoned out. Well, yesterday afternoon it hit me that he still had on the extra patch, so I went and sneaked it off of him. By this morning he was back to normal. Still weak, but cracking jokes and back to his old self (and certainly well enough to tell me how to drive on the trip to the doctor's office!) So, I guess I almost caused him to OD over the weekend! Maybe we need to pray for Keith's protection from ME! Hey, I'm an artist, not a scientist!!

Thank you for all your prayers for today. Please pray that the side effects will be held to a minimum, but most of all that the chemo will do what it was created to do...kill the tumor. He will go each day this week for 5 hours. So glad we are finally underway.

Tuesday, August 11

Day 2 of chemo went good today. They started Keith on Bleomyicin, which is apparently a pretty strong drug. The 5 hour process went fine (he previewed music again), but since we have been home he has begun to feel pretty lousy. He is really fighting with having the hiccups, which apparently is a side effect of the morphine. He has dealt with that this entire time, but it has intensified over the past few days. He also just feels bad, which the doctor had told us to expect.

But, we are getting through this. We are surrounded by the love of a great church, and fabulous friends all over the country. Yesterday we received a "chemo care package" from our dear friends in Ohio. It was full of chemo survival things - everything from chocolate to card games!

Please pray tonight that the side effects will be minimal and that he can rest well. Please pray that the hiccups will cease, but most of all that the tumor is being shrunk. We love you all.

Wednesday, August 12

We are moving along on this interesting road. The chemo went okay today, but it has begun to take a toll on Keith. He is weak and very tired, all of which the doctor told us to expect. He had a little problem with nausea today, but they gave him some medicine and it stopped it. The biggest issue today is that he is retaining a lot of fluid. In the past 3 days he's gained 8 lbs of fluid. His legs are very swollen. They gave him some Lasix today to help with it, and if it is not better tomorrow, he will probably need to see the doctor about it. It's always something!

I feel like we have definitely moved into the marathon portion of this race. It's a long road, but, as Hebrews 12:1 says, "*Therefore, since we are surrounded by such a great cloud of witnesses, let us throw off everything that hinders and the sin that so easily entangles, and let us run with perseverance the race marked out for us.*" This is the race marked out for us, and we are running it (sometimes trudging it!)

Please pray about the fluid retention. They want to get that under control. He also gets the staples out from his surgery tomorrow, which he is not anticipating to be a pleasant experience. But tonight's main prayer request is perseverance as we run this race. Thank you for being the great cloud of witnesses cheering us on!

Thursday, August 13

Well, life rolls along, even when you are dealing with a catastrophic disease! I took Keith to get the surgery staples out this morning, then we headed to chemo. When I came out after getting him set up, my car wouldn't start! Bethany came and got me, then we took cables when we went to pick him up. Poor Keith...5 hours of chemo, then had to come out and jump off my car...THEN go to WalMart and buy a new battery! What a trooper! There are some things that are just "Daddy" things, and I guess buying a car battery is one of those. Wore him out, though...he's sound asleep now!

The fluid buildup was much better today - he had lost 6 lbs. overnight! I tried to get the nurse to give me one of those shots, but she wouldn't do it! They are keeping him on the Lasix since he is getting so much fluid with the chemo. She told him that he is starting to feel the effects of the first days of the chemo, and that it will just compound through next week. Doesn't sound like a very happy week, but at least we are moving forward! The main thing he is experiencing is just being very tired. He has been a little nauseated, but not bad. He also has very little appetite.

Some good news...he is able to go longer now between morphine doses. He was taking it as much as every 2 hours, and yesterday was able to go 4 1/2 hours between doses! The nurse said that the tumor is probably shrinking and pulling off of those nerves. That is a VERY good thing!

Please pray that the side effects will be kept to a minimum, and that the tumor will continue to be obliterated!!!

Friday, August 14

Today there is good news and bad news. First, the bad news is that the side effects of the chemo have really hit Keith. They said it might take a few days for it to kick in, and today it did. He really feels crummy. He made it through the chemo today, and his fluid retention is much better. He has lost 12 lbs of fluid in the last 2 days!

The good news...he went over 7 hours last night without a morphine pill. It wasn't on purpose really, he just decided to try and sleep last night. To put this in perspective, the day he had the surgery and had so many problems with the tumor pain, he had gone 5 hours without a pill, and was literally screaming in pain. I talked with the doctor about it today, and he really feels like the tumor is already shrinking enough that Keith is beginning to feel the difference. He wants me to pull back on the Fentanyl and for him to just use the morphine as he needs it. It is so great to know that this thing is finally starting to respond.

A little funny...I went to get my haircut last night only to discover that my appointment had been for Wednesday evening! And that was after I had changed it twice! Thank goodness for an understanding hairdresser...now I have to wait til next week!! If you see me, remind me that I am getting my hair cut on Wednesday! Too much going on!

I anticipate a rough weekend this weekend. Today Keith said, "Why do I feel so bad?" I responded, "Because you have had 25 hours of poison pumped into your body this week!" I thank God that He has given us a little glimpse that this is working. Please continue to pray for the side effects and for Keith's spirit as he goes through this difficult time.

Monday, August 17

Well, the weekend ended up being as bad or worse than we had thought it might be. Keith was very, very sick the entire weekend. He was very nauseated, and just ached all over. We went back in this morning, for a scheduled visit with the nurse practitioner, and she ended up keeping him for several hours to give him fluids and nausea medicine by IV. As were meeting with her, she kept talking about managing the nausea by Wednesday. Finally I asked why she kept referencing Wednesday, and she said that the drug that Keith is on has a delayed nausea reaction for 5 days, which means by Thursday he should be better! That was fabulous news! At least to me it was...Keith still doesn't believe her!! I thought we were going to be dealing with this nausea stuff for the next 3 months! When I found out it would be over with by Thursday, I told him, "Shoot, I was sick for 4 months during both pregnancies...you can make it another 3 days!!" (Probably not the most sensitive thing to say, now that I think about it.)

So, what we thought would be a 30 min. visit turned out to be a 4 hour stay. That's okay, though, as whatever they gave him has really seemed to help. She said that next week would be his "nourishment week," as he will feel better and needs to strengthen up to do it all again. He can't even think about that right now!

He is off of all the oral morphine, and we have pulled the Fentanyl patch down to 50 mcg, and plan to pull it down to 25 tomorrow night. Getting him off the narcotics has really helped him feel more normal, and to be able to think straight again. He is able to sleep on his side for the first time in months and months. There is no doubt that the chemo has made a difference in the tumor. Hopefully it is still killing it even during the off weeks!

The fluid is also finally gone, and between the loss of fluid and the lack of eating with the nausea, he has lost over 20 lbs. since last week! He's at what would have been his dream weight, but is too sick to enjoy it! I'm sure he will fluctuate some during "nourishment week!" He has lost over 30 lbs since all of this began, and a total of 80 lbs since he first got the lap band!

Several of you have asked about his hair. So far he has not lost any. If it happens, it will probably be this week. Our son has shaved his head in solidarity for his dad. It might be funny if Josh had shaved his head but Keith didn't lose any hair!!

Please pray that, as promised, the nausea will subside by Wednesday, and he can really get his strength back during the next week. Right now he really can't imagine doing this all again in 2 weeks!

Tuesday, August 18

Today was a little bit better for Keith as far as the nausea, but he is so weak and so tired. He had to get another round of the Bleomycin today, and she was telling us that the side effects from that could include headache, low grade fever, and joint pain, so we needed to have Tylenol on hand for tonight. You could see it on poor Keith's face...."Great, now we get to add THOSE things to the mix." He's trying, though. Trying to keep a good attitude. He's just so weak.

In my quiet time yesterday, I read the following passage from Deuteronomy 11:
1. Love the LORD your God and keep his requirements, his decrees, his laws and his commands always. 2.Remember today that your children were not the ones who saw and experienced the discipline of the LORD your God: his majesty, his mighty hand, his outstretched arm; 3. the signs he performed and the things he did in the heart of Egypt, both to Pharaoh king of Egypt and to his whole country; 4. what he did to the Egyptian army, to its horses and chariots, how he overwhelmed them with the waters of the Red Sea as they were pursuing you, and how the LORD brought lasting ruin on them.
5. It was not your children who saw what he did for you in the desert until you arrived at this place, 6. and what he did to Dathan and Abiram, sons of Eliab the Reubenite, when the earth opened its mouth right in the middle of all Israel and swallowed them up with their households, their tents and every living thing that belonged to them. 7. But it was your own eyes that saw all these great things the LORD has done. 8. Observe therefore all the commands I am giving you today, so that you may have the strength to go in and take over the land that you are crossing the Jordan to possess,9. and so that you may live long in the land that the LORD swore to your forefathers to give to them and their descendants, a land flowing with milk and honey.

This may seem like a strange passage to receive comfort from, but it just reminded me again that for over 28 years in ministry, we have had front row seats to the awesome and magnificent works of God in the lives of His people. With tears in my eyes, I sat and reflected on many of the stories that I remember...homes restored, lives put back together, health issues resolved. Many of these stories are your stories...those of you that are reading this and are praying so fervently for us. This passage just reminded me again of the proven dependability of God, and that in these toughest of times we have to pause and remember those times when He showed Himself magnificently. How thankful I am for this truth.

I am claiming verses 8 & 9...Strength to cross over the Jordan, and that land of milk and honey!!

Thank you for indulging me tonight. Thank you for your prayers. We love you all.

Wednesday, August 19

I'll keep today brief, since I have been rather verbose the past couple of days. The news is good...Keith is feeling better! Still really weak, but his color is better and he is feeling stronger. Hopefully this will be the beginning of several days where he feels stronger.

Last night I decided to be Suzy Homemaker and make a homemade chicken pot pie for us for dinner. Well apparently some smell in the recipe really made Keith sick. He couldn't even eat any after smelling it cook! (I ate it...it was good!) So, I have decided that it must not be God's will for me to cook right now....hate that!!! Maybe I'll give it a shot again next week!! Or...maybe not!!

One other cool thing. Many of you know that Josh has started a new job in Dallas. Last week a girl that he works with told him that she is going to run in a half-marathon in October as a fund-raiser for the Lance Armstrong Foundation. She and her family, after hearing Keith's story, are running in honor of him. It is still a fund raiser for the Lance Armstrong Foundation, who had the same kind of cancer as Keith, but they will be honoring Keith as they do it. It meant so much to Josh that one of his friends would do this.

Please pray for continued good days, and strength to get ready for chemo again on the 31st!

Thursday, August 20

Well, it's always something, you know? Today Keith has been doing better from the nausea, but his blood sugar has spiked up. This afternoon it was at 310. A big part of this is our fault, because while he has been so sick, he hasn't taken his regular medications like he was supposed to. SO...we are back on all the pills so hopefully we can get THIS under control. The doctor said that some of the meds that Keith is on could also make it higher.

Because of this and everything else, Keith has really felt bad today. I am really praying that if we can get everything back in line that he can have a good day. We really need a good day.

Please pray that his blood sugar will come down and his energy will go up!

Friday, August 21

Blood sugar is still up, but we did find out today that one of the nausea medications that they give Keith with the chemo has a steroid in it, which can cause the elevated blood sugar. We still have to monitor it and take the meds, but I am glad to know that there was something else at play.

This morning we saw the urologist for his post-surgery visit, and everything is good. In fact he has been released from that doctor. It's GOOD to finally be marking doctors off the list! When we got home this morning, Keith said, "I think I want to go to Peaches." For those non-Bradenton folks, Peaches is a breakfast/lunch diner. We went, and he ate a pretty good bit. It totally wore him out, though, and he went straight to bed when we got home. I was hoping the food might give him a little more energy, but not yet.

I'm hoping he can sleep better tonight. After another bad Ambien experience, the doctor has given Keith Lunesta to help him sleep. We'll see if I have any strange stories about this one!!

He is SO tired and exhausted all the time. I really hope that next week he can bounce back some. We are still looking for that good day. If we have it this weekend, I'll add a special "weekend version." We love you all.

Monday, August 24

Well, finally, a little bit of a positive turn! Keith is feeling a little bit stronger today, and we even went out to lunch! It really wore him out, though, and now he's resting on the couch. That Cracker Barrell is a wild place!

This weekend was rough, but the one thing I know now for sure is that Keith can not take prescription sleep medications. I really think Lunesta was worse for him than the Ambien. Yesterday he was so disoriented when he woke up...then stayed up an hour and went back to sleep. He was literally drugged until yesterday afternoon! So, the strongest thing he can have now is Tylenol PM!

Yesterday was what I call a "wall day." In other words, it was one of those days where I hit a wall with all of this. So many of you have offered sweet prayers for me as the caregiver, and I am so grateful for those, but this wasn't about that. It's not that I am tired or don't want to take care of him...I just miss him. (Okay, I heard that collective, "Awwww!") But it's true. Keith and I share so much and talk so much and he is such a part of me that when we have days like yesterday, I just miss our life and our time together.

He really has no energy. The doctor said that is to be expected, since they have really attacked his immune system and blood count with the chemo. I am hoping now that he is eating a little bit that some of the energy will come back.

Last week I mentioned in one of the posts about a friend of Josh's who has put together a fundraising site for the Lance Armstrong Foundation in honor of Keith. A friend of ours, John Gregory, saw this and is also planning on a half-marathon this fall. He has also put together a site as a fundraiser for Western Indian Ministries, and honoring Keith. For those of you that don't know, Keith has taken mission teams and construction teams to WIM for the past 7 years to help on the Navajo reservation. It is an absolute passion of his. Thanks, guys, for honoring Keith in such a special way!

While today has been a better day, we are still praying for energy for this week. As a friend of our said, "we are praying for a strong, hungry and feeling rejuvenated week!"

Tuesday, August 25

Today's doctor visit revealed that Keith's blood counts are extremely low. His white count is at 1300 with 500 being the infection fighting ones (sorry about my lack of medical knowledge!) Anyway, because it is so low, they decided not to give him the Bleomycin today, and instead gave him another shot to boost his blood count. They are going to do that again tomorrow and then check it again on Thursday. The doctor said that this is why he is experiencing the extreme fatigue. If they can not get the counts up, there is a chance they will postpone the chemo next week, and we really don't want that to happen.

Another milestone today is that he has begun to lose his hair. Even though we knew it was coming, it was a bit of a blow to him to realize it today. This whole cancer journey has new and difficult surprises around every corner!

Please pray that the shots will work and bring his blood count to where it need to be to continue treatment. Also, he lost another 6 lbs. this week, so please pray that his appetite will return and he will be able to eat to gain his strength.

Wednesday, August 26

Hooray! The shot that they have given Keith has really made him feel better. He said earlier that he felt better today than he had in a long time. He got another shot this afternoon, so hopefully he will continue to get stronger!

The big news for today is that I bought clippers at Wal Mart, so we are buzzing his hair tonight! If he'll let me, I'll put a picture on tomorrow! Just be ready, he's lost a lot of weight through his face! I think he's going to look great...and our pastor says he's never going to want to go back to fooling with hair. (For you non-Woodland folks, Tim is completely bald. Check out his Vlog here).

Not much to tell today. It's just good to finally have some good news. AND...Keith has requested that I make his favorite chicken casserole for dinner tonight! So....Suzy Homemaker is back in business!!

Please keep praying about the blood counts. We need to have a white count of at least 2000 before we can move forward.

Thursday, August 27

Yay! Keith's blood counts are up...way up...you guys are good prayer warriors! So glad the shots did what they were supposed to do. So, it looks like he will be set to go to start the next round of chemo on Monday. Never thought THAT would be good news!! The nurse said that now that they know how Keith's body will respond to the chemo, they can do some things differently to hopefully make it easier. Well....we'll see....I think it's gonna be rough no matter what they do!

So how do you like Keith's new hairdo? I think he looks great! both of our kids really like it, too. Bethany said it makes him look 10 years younger! She doesn't want him to go back to the old hairdo! So, maybe we are starting a staff trend....first Tim, then Keith...Andy and Coley, I think you are next!

The bad stuff starts again on Monday, so please begin praying now that it will go as well as it can, but mostly that it is accomplishing the task, and killing the tumor!

Friday, August 28

Keith feels better today than he has in 3 months! Hooray!

I know many of you have walked this road with us, but just for fun, let me do a quick recap....back in the spring, Keith and 2 guys from our church did a Tithe Rap in the service. It required lots of rehearsal and lots of jumping around, and shortly after that, Keith's back started hurting. We all just assumed the back problems were a result of a 50 year old man trying to rap and dance, so he was treated for back pain. As it got worse he had injections to try and block the pain. They thought he had spinal stenosis. SO...he rolled along until the end of June back and forth with the pain better and worse, and in and out of the doctor's office. The first of July it really became unbearable and he started on pain meds.

He got to where he couldn't sleep lying down, so he slept in a chair in our bedroom. As you know, the pain continued to get worse until it reached the pinnacle on July 16 in New Mexico on a Mission Trip, when we flew him home. The next day was the day that will live in infamy...the first day we heard "cancer." Keith went on more potent pain meds until the first week of chemo. After that, the tumor began to shrink and the pain subsided, but the nausea and fatigue took over. **SO...**today is the first day since all of this started that he has been pain-free, off the pain meds, free of nausea, and with a little energy! He's still not ready to run around the block, but he is doing so much better.

The bad news is that Round 2 of the chemo starts on Monday. At least God has given us a glimpse of how things can be after all of this is over. Please pray for next week, and that the side effects will be minimal. He also still is not eating great and needs to try and eat more over the weekend. Thanks for traveling this road with us.

Monday, August 31

Today we started on Round 2 of the chemo. Just like last time, the treatment was pretty uneventful. We know from last time, however, that the icky stuff is coming!

There are a couple of bits of news from the doctor visit today. First, the doctor was VERY excited that Keith was completely off the pain meds. He was thrilled that the tumor has shrunk that much with just one round of chemo. He has scheduled another CT scan for September 16, and depending on what it shows, he'll make the decision whether we are doing 3 or 4 rounds of chemo. Keith is REALLY hoping for 3!

Keith has lost another 4 lbs! He put on a pair of shorts today that some friends brought over (all of his clothes are way too big!) and he is now wearing a waist size that is 10 inches smaller than when he first got the lap band. He's lost 90 lbs. since the lap band! The doctor is not concerned about the weight loss, since Keith is still above recommended weight for someone his height. If he loses much more, though, he said we will have to do something.

He was able to eat a good little bit today, so hopefully he can keep his strength up. Last time when he started the chemo he was so heavily medicated with the pain meds, and he was still recovering from the surgery. Even though he is week this time, I feel like we are starting out with a few more things in our favor.

Any way you look at it, though, it is going to be a rough week, and we so appreciate your prayers. Please pray that we can manage the nausea and that the side effects will be minimal.

Tuesday, September 1

Today the chemo took 6 hours to "infuse!" What a long day! Keith was feeling pretty good afterwards, and asked to go by Kohl's to pick up a few things to wear, since all of his clothes are too big now. This was the first time in 2 months that he has wanted to go somewhere besides the doctor's office, so I said, "sure!" Well, we got into Kohl's and had been there about 10 minutes, and he gave out. So tired he could hardly walk. We managed to pick up a few things, and I stuffed a few things in the basket that we'll try on later, but at least he has underwear, some shorts and a pair of jeans that fit!!

They are giving him more nausea medicine with the chemo this week and I think it is helping him. It's good that they have been able to tailor this week to his needs, now that he has been through it once. He ate a good supper last night and tonight, so I am hoping he will continue to build strength before the side effects really kick in.

Our prayer today is still that the side effects will be minimal, but always that the tumor is shrinking rapidly!

Wednesday, September 2

Today's treatment went without incident. The treat for the day was a visit from some college friends that were passing through town. I took them down to the treatment center, and they visited with Keith for the last hour of his treatment. It was so good to see them, and hear those Alabama accents!

Keith is doing okay this evening, just REALLY tired. He didn't sleep well last night, which they told him is a side effect of the nausea medicine that they are giving through his IV. He's trying to stay awake today so hopefully he can sleep better tonight.

Not much news today, but this is truly a case where no news is good news! Please pray for a good night's sleep tonight for Keith, and for management of the nausea that we feel is looming on the horizon!

Thursday, September 3

We are beginning to realize that "Chemo Thursdays" seem to be our days to have the biggest challenges, and even all out attacks! If you remember our last chemo week, it was on Thursday that my battery died and poor Keith had to jump off the car in the parking lot of the cancer center. Well, this one tops that....boy does it ever!

We got in from chemo today and Keith was really feeling bad. He tried to eat some lunch, and almost immediately got sick. So, he decided to go ahead and lay down in our bedroom. About an hour later, he came to the door of the bedroom and said, "Lee Ann, there's something wrong in here." I jumped up from my desk and went in to find that the toilet had completely backed up and overflowed. There was water and "solid stuff" (gross) all over the floor, all in our shower, and all in the bathtub. I have seen a lot of very gross things, but I have to say...that scene on this day has to rank in the top five of grossness. So, what did I do? I sat down and had a good cry! Not one of those little sniffle cries, I'm talking a good nose-blowing, five-tissue-throwing cry. And you know what, after I finished....all that poop was still there!

When we had the issue with the battery last time, one of the dear men in our church had told me to call him if anything went wrong with the car or house, and he would help us get it fixed. His sweet words were, "Please don't rob me of the blessing to help." So, today, Keith said, "Let's call Brad." He called him, and Brad and his daughter were over here within a half hour. Seeing him on his hands and knees in my shower wiping up the grossest stuff ever, made me wonder if he really regretted that whole "blessing" remark. But what a servant! He called another man in our church who does plumbing, and now Brad and Corky have formed a team to figure out the problem. All the while Keith is laying on the couch trying not to throw up! You can probably imagine that the house is a little "pungent."

Today we have been served by these wonderful people. It was a terrible, icky ordeal, but these folks came in and truly met a need for us. We are blessed and touched by their help and love.

You can pray for our potty tonight, but I think we are in good hands with Corky and Brad. Please do pray for Keith as he finishes the chemo. He's really entering into the rough stuff.

Friday, September 4

Well, the full force of the chemo experience has now surrounded Keith. He's got the fatigue and the nausea, and can hardly hold his head up. We've been through before, though, and now that we know the routine, we know it is just a matter of getting through it. One of the things he is looking forward to is the return of College Football this weekend, specifically Alabama Football! If anything can get him involved and yelling, it will be watching his beloved Crimson Tide! In fact, I don't ever think I have seen him watch an Alabama football game without yelling, so maybe this will be the medicine that he needs!

All of our plumbing is running well today. The events of yesterday have put me in a house cleaning mood, so I've been scrubbing and reorganizing, and plan to continue through the weekend. Just have to be careful that none of my cleaning stuff smells make Keith sick! If that happens, then guess I'll just have to stop!!

Thank you for your prayers during this difficult Chemo week. Please continue to pray about the side effects and the delayed effects that he won't even experience until next week. Also, please pray now for the CT Scan on the 16th. How wonderful would it be if they looked at the scan and couldn't even find the tumor! Even if we can't have that, we are praying for just one more round of chemo.

Monday, September 7

Keith is very sick today. He is nauseated, but mostly overwhelmingly fatigued. It's just like last time, which brings me a little comfort in knowing that he is traveling the same path. He is surviving on Propel, popsicles, and a little bit of soup. That's okay, though. We just need to get through it. Things should get better by Wednesday.

We see the doctor tomorrow, and he is supposed to get more chemo and a shot that will boost his blood count. I just want everything to stay on track, so we can keep moving toward the goal.

Tuesday, September 8

Today was a little bit better as far as the sickness. Keith was not nearly as nauseated, but still is dealing with the terrible fatigue. We went to the doctor today, and he got the Bleomyicin. His blood counts were a little low, but not terrible. We go back tomorrow and he is supposed to get a shot that will really boost his blood count and hopefully give him some more energy.

Please be praying for the results that we will see next week (Sept. 16) on the CT Scan. We are really praying that the tumor has shrunk drastically. Please also pray for his energy level. He is so wiped out.

Sorry I'm not very chatty tonight, but between work, doctor, and 2 pharmacy runs, I am beat. More tomorrow!

Wednesday, September 9

Today started out promising, as Keith was up doing odds and ends and reading his email this morning. After he finished, though, it was like the bottom dropped out of his energy level, and he was done!

We went to the doctor this afternoon and he got a Neulasta shot, which is supposed to boost his immune system and his blood count. Last time the shots helped the extreme fatigue, so we are hoping that it will have the same effect this time. He is just so wiped out, and really is not himself because he is so tired.

We have now completed 31 days of what we hope will be a 54 day ordeal (since he began treatment). If the doctor adds a fourth round of chemo, then I guess our days will stretch to 75. Whatever the amount, 75 days out of our lives is not overwhelming. It's a little difficult when you are standing in the middle of it, but we are going to get through it.

Thank you for all of your kind emails. It is truly amazing and humbling to know there are people all over the country, many that we have never met, that are praying for us. Please know that we never take that for granted, and I am so thankful that you care enough to lift our names to the Father. You have blessed us.

Thursday, September 10

This morning Keith got up and was feeling good. He had a speakerphone call from Tim and the Woodland staff, as they were at an all day long planning meeting and wanted him to know that they missed him. They prayed for him, and it really meant a lot to him that they had called. He had spent all yesterday afternoon getting his dates ready for the meeting, and Andy was supposed to fight for his dates!

I was really singing the praises of Neulasta this morning, even had Keith and I cast in a Neulasta commercial in my mind....but, alas, about lunch time he started getting sick. He's still better than he has been, but he spent most all afternoon on the couch. I wish we could get the whole digestive thing figured out. Tonight he had applesauce and mashed potatoes. I am really praying that he will just continue to get stronger since we have all of next week before we have to start it all over again.

We are going to shave his head again tomorrow. His nubby hair has started growing out some, and today I told him he had "chemo hair." I guess that wasn't the most sensitive thing to say, so now he's after me to shave it again.

Please continue to pray for regained strength for him and that he will be able to eat. We love you all.

Friday, September 11

Today has been a good day! While Keith still doesn't have a tremendous amount of energy, he did a few things around the house today, and even walked the dog! It is so good to see him up and around. He's still surviving on soup and Propel, but at least he's not sick.

Our prayer requests for this weekend: 1. That his blood count will stay up. Last time it was over this weekend that they dropped so low and he felt so bad. 2. That the CT Scan will reveal that the treatment is working and that we hopefully won't have to do the 4th round. 3. That he will continue to get stronger before he has to enter into Round 3!

Thank you for your prayers.

Monday, September 14

Keith is doing very well today! He is up and going, even in working on Woodland stuff right now.

The weekend was a bit challenging, however. The Neulasta shot that I was so high on last week has some interesting side effects. Apparently your body produces white blood cells in your lower back/pelvic region. The Neulasta causes an extreme increase in this production. They had told us that he might have some pain associated with this, and boy did he ever! It started on Friday evening and got progressively worse until I finally called the doctor yesterday. He said that it is not unusual for Neulasta to cause that, and wanted to know if we had any pain medicine (this was not our doctor, but one of the other doctors on call). I laughed and said, "We've got pretty much anything you want him to take!" He decided on the 30 mg. of morphine. It took care of the pain, but knocked Keith FLAT! It's interesting that he at one time was taking that every 3 hours! Anyway, the pain has eased up some now and he hasn't had any of the morphine since 4 this morning. So hopefully we are past the really rough part of it.

Our Sunday morning ritual has pretty much gone like this for the past month or so: First, at 9 am we come in here to the computer and watch the Woodland live streaming of the service. After that, Keith usually goes into the living room and watches Ed Young or some other minister that he finds on TV. Then he will usually turns on GMT. This past weekend there was a Gaither broadcast on GMT. I was in at the computer, and I heard him saying, "Amen...amen!" I went in, and David Phelps was singing the chorus to "These are They." Tears were streaming down Keith's face as he raised his hands in worship. For those of you unfamiliar with the song, these are the lyrics:

These are they
Who have come out of great tribulation
They have washed their robes in the blood of the Lamb
They have come through much sorrow into great jubilation
They're redeemed by the blood of the Lamb[1]

Songs like that have taken on new meaning after the journey of the past few months. I believe with all my heart that Keith's passion as a worship leader will be stronger and more annointed as a result of coming through this tribulation period. We're both just ready to be there!

Tuesday, September 15

What a crazy day. It started out pretty well. Keith was feeling weak, but okay. He had a visit from some of the ladies from the office, just wanted to come by and visit. He enjoyed that, but it really tired him out more than usual. So, we then went to the doctor for his Tuesday treatment (Bleomyicin). Even that went fine.

But when we got home, things went into a downward spiral. He went straight in and got into bed, and he began shivering and complaining that he was freezing. I got more blankets for him and felt of him to be sure he wasn't running fever, and he wasn't. I let him sleep, then woke him up about 7 pm. The Navajo Mission Trip group was getting together for dinner tonight, so I told him that I was heading out for that. When I got back just before 9, he was sitting on the couch and told me he really didn't feel good. He was disoriented and couldn't get his thoughts together, which really concerned me. I reached over and felt of him, and he was burning up! I took his temp and it was 102!

I called the doctor, and luckily the doctor on call was our oncologist, and he said he is sure that Keith has an infection. He called in an antibiotic for me to get him started on and wants to run some tests on him in the morning. He has postponed the scan until Thursday. He told me that if the fever gets higher or if he gets sicker that he wants to put him in the hospital. Boy, on this journey, you never know what's around the next bend!

Please pray that the antibiotic will take care of the infection, and that the tests will help them know what it is. The doctor thinks he might have colitis, an infection of the colon. Keith really wants to have the CT scan done, so please pray that we can have it done on Thursday. Thank you for rallying around us...I already feel your strength.

Wednesday, September 16

Well, Keith's fever has been down all day today, and we are hoping that whatever caused is being taken care of by the antibiotics. He had to go in today to for a couple of tests. They think he might have a urinary infection or colitis, so he had to provide some "gifts" for them! We haven't heard anything on that yet. They have moved the CT Scan to Friday. That means we won't have the results by Monday, but the doctor said that no matter what the results are, we will be doing the 3rd round.

Keith has felt good all day today. We even went to lunch with our Worship Associate and Tech Director today. He didn't eat much, but surely enjoyed the time to visit. He is planning on going to the Worship Arts Kickoff tomorrow night, and will be leading in part of the services this weekend. Of course, after the events of yesterday we have learned that our plans can change quickly!

I am hoping for a calm evening tonight! Thank you again for all of your prayers and emails.

Thursday, September 17

The Cancer Center called this morning to let us know that Keith's Magnesium count was very low, and the doctor wanted him to come in for a Magnesium drip. SO, we loaded up and headed down there this afternoon. They told him that it should make him feel better, and it really did. I think that treatment really helped him be able to do all he did tonight.

Tonight was the Worship Arts Ministry Kickoff, and Keith felt well enough to go and make an appearance. I couldn't hold back the tears when he walked in the room and it erupted in cheers! He did a great job speaking and challenging the group. He was stronger than I have see him in a long time, and he looked great in his "skinny" jeans! The Worship Arts team gave us a WONDERFUL scrapbook full of memories from our last 4 years. We missed our 4 year anniversary (August 22), so this was their recognition and gift. It is so special, as each of our team members did a page.

We have the CT Scan at 10 am in the morning. Keith has to drink the gross barium drink starting at 7 am. Please pray that he can get it all down and that the test will go okay. Most of all we are praying that the test will show that the tumor has shrunk even more than they had hoped.

Friday, September 18

Keith has felt better today than he has in a long time. He got up this morning and drank the icky barium drink and we headed out for the CT Scan. That was a little rough, as they had to stick him 8 times before they could get the IV in for the contrast! He looked like a pin cushion! Then, he had to go back to the cancer center to give blood for them to test the magnesium levels. The nurse there said he was especially "holely" today! It was so good to hear him joking with the nurses. It's like he was back to his old self.

After all the medical stuff, we went out for breakfast, and had a great day. I know that round 3 of the chemo is lurking around the corner, but today was such a nice gift!

He will start Round 3 of the chemo on Monday. We hope it is the last round. We should know that sometime next week. He is still planning on participating in the services this weekend. Please pray for him, as I know Sunday especially will be tiring for him since there are 2 services. Remember if you would like to watch him, you can log on to our live streaming at www.woodlandlive.com. Services are Saturday at 5 pm and

Sunday at 9 & 10:45 am (ET). he probably won't be on until about 10-15 minutes into the service.

Monday, September 21

What a great weekend we had! Keith led worship in all 3 services. Tim brought him out at the welcome and gave him a different Harley dew rag at each service! It was so good to see him back on the platform, and the response of our people was wonderful.

So, we got good news and bad news at the doctor today. The good news is really good. The tumor has shrunk to 1/3 of its original size. The volume of the tumor was 20" when we started, and now it is 8". Here's what the report said, for all you medical types out there: "Quite massive periaortic retroperitoneal adenopathy has significantly diminished in size with the shape of the conglomerate mass of nodes remaining roughly similar to the prior study, although the overall volume is markedly diminished." Don't you feel smart?! The doctor is very pleased with this information and the progress.

Now, the bad news. He said we would have to do the 4th round of chemo. It was pretty sad news for a bit, but then we realized that finally we could pu an ending date on this thing. Keith will have chemo this week, will be sick next week, and then recover the week after that. He will start the final round of chemo on October 12. So we will be completely through with chemo by October 16. That means today marked the passing of the halfway point. We have completed 11 days, and have 9 more to go of chemo!

The weekend really restored Keith's passion. When we were on the way home on Sunday, he said, "I could go back and do 3 more services!" He took his laptop to chemo today and did some work, and made phone calls and plans now that he knows what the future looks like.

Even with all this good news, we know that we are entering a chemo week, which means lots of fatigue and sickness. Please pray for this week and the effects on his body. Also, he is very anemic. They are going to give him a Procrit shot tomorrow, but if that doesn't raise his red blood count, they will have to do a transfusion. We really don't want that. Please pray for improved blood counts. Chemo just wreaks havoc on all parts of your body! But...9 more days of treatment to go!!

Tuesday, September 22

Today's treatment was relatively uneventful. Keith was really dreading going this morning. By now we know what the week is going to be like, and it is difficult to move forward knowing what is around the corner!

It really stinks because he was doing so well on Sunday, but then as the chemo starts doing its thing, he starts to fade.
Today when we came in he almost immediately fell asleep on the couch, and then moved into the bedroom. It really wipes him out. Today was also the Bleomyicin, which usually gives him a low-grade fever.

It's all part of it. I don't know whether it's better to know what's coming, or to just roll along in ignorance! But either way, we are doing fine...moving along now that the end is in site!

I have received many emails from those of you who enjoyed watching the video. Sorry we had technical issues with some of the services this weekend. Join us again this weekend. Keith won't be there, but we'll be watching online!

Today the biggest prayer request is still the red blood count. He got a Procrit shot today, so we are really hoping that will boost it up. I will keep you posted!

Wednesday, September 23

Chemo is such an awful thing. While I know if is beneficial in the long run, it absolutely sucks the life and energy out of Keith. I guess this is the first time it has happened right before my eyes. He was so strong and vibrant last weekend, then little by little as he has been in treatment this week, he has gotten weaker. Still not sick, but very tired and weak.

This week has been difficult for both of us. I think primarily because of the high we were on after the weekend. It was so awesome to see him back leading in worship. Then Monday morning we had to start over! Every day gets us closer to the end, though.

Still no word on the blood count. They didn't check it today. Keep praying about that. I am sure that they will check it tomorrow or Friday. And more than likely the sickness will really hit him tomorrow. Please pray that it will be managed and pass quickly.

Tomorrow is another "chemo Thursday" (*scary music inserted here*). So far "chemo Thursdays" have brought dead batteries and backed up toilets. I know you will wait with anticipation to see what interesting story I have to tell tomorrow!

Thursday, September 24

We have managed to come through "Chemo Thursday" virtually unscathed! No major events, and for that I am extremely thankful.

This has been a really rough week for us. I described it to a friend today as when you take a beach ball and you pull out the air plug and it slowly deflates. That's how it has been watching Keith as this week has gone on. He has gotten weaker and weaker. We knew it would happen...we've done this three times now, but the contrast between last weekend and now is so stark.

A group of Keith's peers really ministered to him today. He is a member of a group of 50 Music Ministers from all over the country called Metro II. They email ideas and questions back and forth to each other throughout the year, and then meet together for a conference in February. All the churches are similar in size and they are always a great support to each other for resources and ideas.

Today, one of the men sent out an email encouraging all the Metro guys to watch the video of Keith leading worship. He received many encouraging and uplifting emails from these guys. Keith had taken his phone with him to chemo today (which he usually doesn't), so he was able to get the emails as they came in. He couldn't even tell me about it without tears. They really ministered to him at a time when he really needed it. I am so thankful that God sent that ray of light into a pretty bleak week. Thanks, Metro guys!!

The nausea and fatigue have started, and we will have a long weekend. At least Alabama's on TV this weekend, so he can get his football fix! We have a new stash of nausea pills, so please pray that they work! Also, one of the chemo drugs has a steroid in it, and it is causing him to be unable to sleep at night. Please pray for a restful night tonight. He has also begun to have the metallic taste in his mouth that so many have mentioned. That's a new thing, and he hates it! Hopefully it will subside as soon as the chemo is over.

We have reached the point of just putting one foot in front of the other. It's a tough part of the journey, but we feel your support and prayers.

Friday, September 25

We have completed another Chemo week and it is already taking its toll. Keith has all the usual maladies: nausea, fatigue, diarrhea, and just overall feeling like he's been hit by a bus.

As I mentioned before, this has been a hard week, and I'm glad to see it done! We will hunker down for the weekend...eat a lot of soup, watch a lot of football, and take a lot of naps. Wow! I remember when that used to sound like a great weekend! Everything is relative!

Thank you for your prayers. Please continue to pray for his blood counts. They will check them again on Tuesday. Also, please pray that we can manage all of these side effects and that the "bounce back" will happen quickly.

Monday, September 28

Well, as Chemo Weekends go, this one wasn't too bad. At least Friday and Saturday were pretty good. Keith was tired, but overall felt okay, and was even able to eat a little. But, the wrath of chemo came in on Sunday morning and is still with us. He has spent all day today either in the bed or on the couch, and really feels bad. The only up side is that we know it will get better as the week goes on.

I have to wonder if his blood counts are off again since he is so weak. We see the doctor tomorrow, and they will decide based on his blood counts what to do next. He may get the Neulasta shot again, and he will probably get another Procrit shot. (Neulasta for white blood cells, Procrit for red blood cells).

We were talking over the weekend about life after chemo, and all the things we wanted to do. Keith said, "I just want to feel normal again and do normal things. I'm really looking forward to just getting up and going in to the office!" Dear ones out there...don't take those simple things in your life for granted!! The one thing we have learned is that things can change very quickly!

Tuesday, September 29

The fun twists and turns on this ride just keep coming! As I suspected, Keith's blood counts were low. I just had no idea how low! They even re-drew the blood to be sure it was right! For those of you that know about such things, his red count is just below 7, his white count is at .9, and his neutrofils are at 500. So, he got a Neulasta and Procrit shot today, and he has to go to the hospital tomorrow for a blood transfusion. It's certainly not what we were planning for, but at this point in the ride, we just have to continue to trust.

He has been put on "house arrest" for the next few days, until the shots and the transfusion begins to work, as his body right now has nothing to fight off infection. The doctor has started him on an antibiotic just to help fight any infection. They said in the next few days he would definitely begin to feel better, and would probably feel a good bit better after the transfusion.

Today was really bad as far as the nausea and fatigue. Keith couldn't even hardly get out of bed. So, I am really hoping that all of the stuff that they are doing will strengthen him. Boy...are we ever ready to be done with this!!

Please pray for the transfusion tomorrow. Pray that it will go without incident, and that it will do what they hope. Also please pray that all the shots and stuff that they have given him will boost his counts. Please pray that he will have a bubble of protection around him as he goes into the hospital tomorrow to protect him from any infection.

Finally, please pray for our spirits. All this stuff just zaps the life out of both of us. I really understand the scripture in Isaiah 40:31: "But those who hope in the Lord shall renew their strength. They shall mount up with wings like eagles, they shall run and not grow weary, they shall walk and not faint." I'm learning that the walking without fainting is really more difficult than flying like an eagle. But our hope is in the Lord, so we will walk and not faint. We'll get back to the flying stuff later.

Wednesday, September 30

Well, Keith is all pumped full of new blood! He had his "blood transplant" this morning. They gave him 2 units. We had a lot of fun on the way down this morning speculating on whose blood he was getting...girl blood or boy blood, maybe somebody with curly hair so he would grow a headful of hair! Okay, I had fun speculating, Keith wasn't in any shape to enjoy anything! He did perk up a little when they started the transfusion. As the blood slowly started making its was through the tube toward his body he kept saying, "freaky!" I think everyone in the room realized that he was the blood rookie!

The transfusion seems to have helped. Now that he has had the shots and the blood, he has all the tools, we just have to wait for his body to respond. Our prayer request for today is just that it will all work, and those counts will come back up. Also, he had a lot of pain with the Neulasta before (it causes pain in the lower back and legs as it makes the new bone marrow), so please pray that it will be minimal this time. What a journey!

Thursday, October 1

Keith is doing a little better today. Well, I guess he is doing a lot better since Tuesday, but he still is really wiped out. He poked around the house a little today, but it really wore him out. It is amazing how this particular week in the treatment can fluctuate so drastically from one round to the next.

There's really not a lot of news today. We are still waiting for everything to fully "kick in" so he will hopefully keep getting stronger and stronger....and then we get to do it all over again....but just one more time!!

Friday, October 2

Keith is getting stronger every day, for which I am so thankful! He is still pretty weak today, but definitely better than yesterday and light years from Wednesday before the transfusion.

We have our close friends, Paul and Mariann Strozier here for the weekend, and we have both very much been looking forward to it. Paul has been a pastor to us for over 15 years, and it is great to have the time with them. They are true friends...perfectly content to sit with us in our pajamas and watch Alabama football (even though they are Georgia fans)!!

Please pray that the strengthening will continue and we won't hit anymore bumps in the road next week. Keith is scheduled to lead worship next weekend, and he really is hoping he will be able to do it.

Monday, October 5

This weekend was wonderful - we had our friends, the Stroziers here, which really lifted Keith's spirits. They got up Saturday morning and cleaned our house from top to bottom! I protested, but they didn't listen...they saw what needed to be done and did it. I'm really learning a lot about servanthood through this process, and Paul and Mariann are true servants. After the marathon cleaning, Paul sat with Keith through the Alabama game, the Georgia game, and the Auburn game!

The good news is that Keith is really feeling stronger. We went to the beach for an hour or so yesterday. Most of you know what a beach bum Keith is, and he has not been to the beach since June! (For those of you that don't know, we live about 30 min. from the coast.) He LOVED being back at the beach, even though he didn't have the energy to do much more than sit! And the trip wore him out!

Today has been good. He gets up and putters around the house until he is wiped out, then comes back to the couch. At least he is not sick, though. We go to the doctor tomorrow for more bloodwork and a round of Bleomyicin. Unless we hit another roadblock, he should continue to get stronger as the week goes on. Please join us in praying for that. He is planning on leading worship in the services this weekend. Then, a week from today we will start the FINAL round!

Tuesday, October 6

Well, I always wonder if the day will come when I really have nothing to write on here. No such luck today! You know how I mentioned roadblocks yesterday? Well, today Keith has felt good. He's had pretty good energy and no sickness. We went to the doctor for his appointment and they did the usual bloodwork. Shock to us all, his red count was back down to 7 again, and his white count was low, too. The biggest thing, though, is that his platelets were at 15,000. Last week they were at 300,000, and normal is 100,000-400,000. SO...they wouldn't even let us come home. They sent him straight to the hospital for platelets. He has to go back tomorrow for another blood transfusion.

I learned comething about Chemo today. The damage that it does to both the bad cells and the good is cumulative. It is still in there killing stuff when he starts the next round of chemo, and the new chemo just joins the old. So, the battle of the next few weeks will be with these blood counts. We need to keep them up and get him through the final treatment so he can begin to heal from all of it. Again today they told us that once he completes the treatment all of this will come back to normal, but we have to keep him healthy and free of infection until then.

Needless to say, today's prayer request has to do with blood counts and transfusions and protection from infection. If the counts don't come back up, he will have to hold off a week on the final chemo. We have to go back for bloodwork on Thursday. I really thought this was going to be an uneventful week!!

Wednesday, October 7

Keith received 2 units of blood today and seems to feel stronger. I don't know, he was feeling pretty good before he went, but he says he feels better! They are checking his blood again tomorrow, and if it is still low, we may have to go in for more on Friday

Bethany came in today for the weekend, and it is so good to have her home. She hasn't seen Keith since he started chemo, but she really likes the no hair look! I know she will keep us entertained this weekend!

Please join me in praying about these blood counts. This is a really big deal, and could keep him from starting the final round of chemo. We really don't want that to happen. While we are not looking forward to next week, we are really looking forward to what it represents...the FINAL week!!

Thursday, October 8

Hooray! The counts are back up! It seems that the Neulasta has kicked in, and the transfusion has done its thing, so they were very pleased at the doctor's office today! His platelets still are not where they need to be, but he's out of the red zone, so we are happy with that. We'll just be sure to keep him away from sharp objects!

We had a visit today from some longtime friends, Eddy and Mary McBroom. Eddy and Keith served on staff together for many years in Birmingham, and it was great fun to see them. Eddy and Keith had many big laughs about antics from those days! Eddy was Bethany's first youth minister and he and Mary have always been special to her, so she also really enjoyed seeing them.

Please continue to pray about the blood counts. Also, Keith received the Bleomyicin today, which always makes him feel a little rough. He is still planning on the weekend services...please pray God's protection around him!

Friday, October 9

Keith went to church last night to do the run through with the band and choir for the weekend. He so enjoyed being there, but he was completely tuckered out when we got home! Also, the Bleomyicin causes him to run a low grade fever, so he had that to deal with as well last night.

Today, however, has been good. He hasn't had a lot of energy, but he has felt good and has really enjoyed having Bethany home. They have a big football-watching day planned for tomorrow. Auburn plays at noon, then Alabama is at 3:30. Of course, Keith has to be at the church at 3:30, so he will tape it and watch it when we get home. He just avoids anyone who might know the outcome before we get home! I'm sure they will watch the FLA/LSU game tomorrow night.

I keep thinking that this time next week we will be all the way through with the chemo. I can't imagine that, and I can't wait!! Please pray that we will continue on without any setbacks. We love you all.

Monday, October 12

Well....POOH!! We went to the doctor today all set to begin the final week of this blessed experience, only to find that the doctor has postponed it a week. We begged, but he really wants Keith to have another week for his blood to recover before we do it all again. His counts were good, but still a little low, and the doctor is afraid that they would really bottom out if we decided to move forward. So, while we are really ready to get it over with, it is nice to know that we will have another week where he should feel pretty good. Shoot...he even says he's taking me out to dinner tonight!!

He was making his list of things he wants to accomplish this week as we were on our way home from the cancer center. I think he's even planning on a day or two at the office! We'll see...his goals may be a little bigger than his energy level.

He did a great job this weekend in worship, and he so enjoyed being back doing what he loves. He didn't have quite the energy that he had last time, but the doctor said that is also because of the anemia.

We go in for a Procrit shot tomorrow, and then nothing else until next Monday. Please pray that the counts keep coming up!

Tuesday, October 13

Keith had a good day today. In fact, he DROVE himself to the cancer center to get his shot. That is the first time since he entered the hospital on July 17 that he has driven a car! When he got out of the hospital he was on morphine and couldn't drive, and since he has started treatment he has been too weak. It was sort of funny...I made him call me when he got there just to be sure he got there okay! Just like I used to do with our kids when they first started driving!

We did go out to eat last night - it was great! So glad to be doing some normal things. I think he is even going in to the office tomorrow.

They did bloodwork on him today and the counts were up a little. Hopefully they will continue moving upward so that we can get this final week of treatment behind us! Please continue to pray about the blood counts!

Wednesday, October 14

Today brought more activity and strength. Keith went in to the office this morning and stayed for our Worship Planning meeting. Then we went out to lunch with some of the Worship Arts team...it was a great day! However, his energy level isn't back to normal...he came home and slept for two hours!

This week has really been a gift. I do have to remind myself that we have to go back into the black hole next week, but this week has reminded me that we will emerge from this! I know the recovery will be slow, but it is so good to see him every day getting stronger. Hopefully his blood is responding and getting stronger, too.

The main thing I want to seek your prayers about is protection from all the "bugs" that are around. We have lots of cases of swine flu and regular flu in our schools. Once he starts back on the chemo, we will sequester away, but I would appreciate your prayers of protection.

Thursday, October 15

Well, I'm thinkin' Keith may have overdone it a little this week. He was REALLY tired all day today. I'm hoping it is the fact that he has done too much, and not a dip in the blood counts that has made him tired. He took a long nap, and felt a little better after that.

He did the rehearsal tonight, and before we went he said, "I really hope I can do this." He wanted me to park close to the door and to be ready to leave as soon as rehearsal was over. I know most of you are surprised, but I do tend to talk a little after rehearsal. The interesting thing is that he seemed stronger during the rehearsal, and after it was over he said, "It was like the rehearsal re-energized me. I felt stronger and stronger as it went on. " I guess that is the power of praising God!!

Please continue to pray about his blood counts. We are really hoping to be almost through with this a week from now.

Friday, October 16

Still not a lot of energy today. Keith tried to tackle the project of pulling all the oversized clothes from his closet. I think he was a little surprised at the amount of XXL clothes that he owns! At one point he tried on a long sleeved XXL oxford-type shirt, and it swallowed him whole! The shoulders came halfway down his arm! Anyway, he tuckered out about halfway through the project, so I guess we'll have to fold up some shirts before we can go to bed tonight!

We went out to dinner with some great friends tonight, and he did great and really enjoyed it. It's funny that the blessing he prays at meals now includes the phrase, "please help me eat it, digest it, and keep it down" and he means it!

Please continue to pray about the blood counts. Keith is doing the services this weekend, so please pray for energy for that. We are really hoping to start the final round on Monday. Please join us in that prayer. We are ready to ring the chemo graduation bell!!

Monday, October 19

Hooray! We started the last round of chemo today! I am SO glad that all the bloodwork was okay so he could move forward. So, we have this week of chemo, then he will be sick this weekend and next week. The week of November 2 he will begin the recovery process. He has to go back each week for bloodwork until November 16, which is when we have the scans scheduled. Then, November 19, a month from today, we have our appointment with the doctor to go over the scans. There's a light at the end of the tunnel!

Last night Keith realized that he has lost all of his bottom eyelashes and most of his top ones. You don't realize how important those little guys are until you don't have them! He also no longer has to shave. He hasn't shaved in over 2 months. I guess that will make the "upside of chemo" list.

Thank you so much for your prayers. Just please continue to pray for strength and protection during this final round.

Tuesday, October 20

Today went pretty well. Keith has had a new nurse at the Cancer Center for the past two days, and because she is new, his treatment is taking longer. Today he was there for just over 6 hours. That's a LONG day! AND they gave him Lasix to help with the fluid retention, so he was back and forth to the bathroom every 30 min!

He hasn't been sick yet, just very tired. He took a long nap today, and when he woke up he decided he wanted a pressed Cuban sandwich from a sandwich shop down the road. I went and got it, thinking there was no way he would eat it, but when I got home he ate every bite!

Please pray about the side effects of the treatment. There is so much going on in his body. We are just ready for this to be done!

Wednesday, October 21

It is amazing to me how similar, yet how different each round of the chemo has been. This time (so far), Keith has not been sick. He has had a good appetite and is able to eat. He has, however, had overwhelming fatigue. He had his regular nurse today, so the chemo went faster, but by the time he got home he was SO tired.

Of course the fatigue is bad, but if the nausea will stay away, his life will be so much easier over the next few days. I forgot to mention, though, that although he is very tired, he is having insomnia at night thanks to a steroid that they are giving him through the chemo. So he just sleeps at weird times, whenever he can! Winnie (our dog) is always ready to keep him company for a nap!

Two more days...so ready for him to ring that chemo graduation bell!

Thursday, October 22

Keith came home from chemo today completely wiped out. As I write this, he has been asleep for over 2 1/2 hours. I am glad of this, as he is not sleeping well at all at night. Last night he was up every hour.

One more day of the 5-hour chemo!! They told him he won't ring the chemo bell until he completes the last Bleomyicin (the short chemo that he gets on Tuesdays). That will be week after next. Bell or no bell, we will be cheering as we leave the center tomorrow! He will go next Tuesday for Bleo and bloodwork, the same on the following Tuesday, and then have the scans on November 16. We are praying that when they do the scans they will find no remnant of that big tumor!

Chemo Thursday has once again been uneventful, thank goodness! Please pray that as the chemo goes through his body that the side effects will be minimal.

Friday, October 23

HOORAY! The last day of chemo is over!! I know there are still lots of things that we will have to do, but at least the consecutive days of sitting in that chair for 5-6 hours are over! We figured out today that he has had over 100 hours of chemo. That doesn't even include the blood transfusions or the Magnesium drips that he has had!

It's like we are both scared to say it out loud that he is through with chemo. With every step of this there have been unexpected twists and turns, so I guess we are both just waiting for the doctor to say...."You are really through!" Maybe it will feel more real when he rings the Chemo Graduation Bell on November 2!

He is still VERY fatigued, and has started with a little nausea this afternoon. Hopefully we can keep it at bay with the medicine, and just focus on helping him get stronger now that this part is over.

Please pray about his blood counts. That will be the real critical thing over the next week or so.

You know, I said at the beginning of this that we were in a marathon. If you are still reading this every day, then you have run the marathon with us, and you will never know this side of Heaven what your faithful friendship, prayers and emails have meant to us. We're in the final stretch, we hope!

Monday, October 26

The full effects of the chemo did not hit Keith until yesterday, so he had a pretty good evening on Friday, and felt pretty good on Saturday, he was just VERY tired. Of course, when Alabama blocked the last second field goal that would have cost them the game, you should have seen him come up off the couch! Of course, shortly after that, he was ready for bed! I think all the excitement wore him out.

Yesterday about mid-morning he began to really feel bad, and has been feeling rough ever since. We go tomorrow for bloodwork and Bleomyicin, so please pray with us that his blood counts will stay strong. He is so wiped out that I am concerned that they may be dropping again.

It really hasn't hit us that the long chemo sessions are over with. Or maybe we won't let our guard down until we actually get the results of the scans. Whatever, we are just taking it a day at a time, trying to focusing on getting him stronger and moving back toward life beyond cancer!

Tuesday, October 27

The icky sick of the chemo has arrived. He is not real nauseated, but really has no energy and just feel awful. We went in today for bloodwork and his counts were actually pretty good. His white count was a little low, but otherwise he was good. They gave him the Bleomyicin today. Just one more treatment!!

We were talking last night about how we can't believe it is already the end of October. In some ways it seems like we are still stuck in July. I have picked up most of Keith's prescriptions at the Walgreen's across the road from us. When I first started, their center aisle had beach buckets and flip flops, and I was picking up morphine for his pain. Then we moved into nausea management and the center aisle had turned into back to school stuff. More recently the center aisle has been fall and Halloween, and I noticed yesterday when I was picking up the latest prescription (for thrush in his mouth), that they had started putting the Christmas stuff out. I hope this is the last holiday we get to celebrate with them!

We go in tomorrow for Neupagin shots to boost his white count. Please pray for continued strength and for his blood counts. He just need to continue to get stronger and stronger. And, of course, please pray for the scans on November 16. We are praying that the tumor and any hint of the cancer will be gone!

Wednesday, October 28

Today has been a rough day. Keith felt pretty good this morning, in fact he felt good enough for us to meet some friends for lunch. After lunch, however, his energy level began to drop. We went to the Cancer Center today for the shot that is supposed to help his blood count, and by the time we got home he was so tired he could hardly hold his head up. He slept for awhile, but was still tired after he woke up. We go back for another shot tomorrow, and I think if he is still this tired tomorrow I'm going to call ahead and see if they will check his blood.

I peeked in on him while he was sleeping today, and he looked so frail in the bed. I know he will continue to get stronger, but this has been such a long journey, and we are ready for the turn. He has lost all of his eyelashes and most of his eyebrows. He has virtually no muscle tone in his arms and legs. Chemo really does wreak havoc on the body. But thankfully we have one more treatment and then he can ring the graduation bell!

Please continue to pray about the counts. We are ready for another good day!

Thursday, October 29

I had to write a little earlier today to let you know that Keith is really having a good day today. After I wrote the entry last night, we realized that Keith was running a fever of around 100.5. When we got that down he started feeling better, and he slept better last night. Today he has felt much stronger.

I know my entry sounded pretty sad last night, and to be honest, even this late in the process, I was pretty sad. I still have those "wall" days, where I just feel like I have hit a wall with all of this. God is gracious, though, to help pick me up and get me out of the pity party mode and help me realize how blessed we are.

So, thanks for allowing me to be transparent, and thanks for all of your sweet emails, and know that your prayers are being answered, both for Keith and for me.

Keith is planning on driving himself down to get his shot today, so look out Bradenton drivers...Keith Martin will be on the loose!

Friday, October 30

Wow, what a difference 48 hours (and your prayers) can make! Keith is feeling really good today. He even drove himself to the church and did a little straightening in his office. It is SO good to see him up and around...right now he is sitting at the kitchen table checking emails on his laptop.

He got a really nice email yesterday from a local man who has just come through treatment for testicular cancer. This fellow met a friend of ours down in St. Pete, and Greg asked him to contact Keith when he found out that he had already completed the treatment. His email was so encouraging to Keith. He told him to hang in there and that he would be surprised how quickly his energy would come back once he was through with the treatments. We have met lots of people with lots of different cancer through this process, but this man is the first one that had the same type of cancer that Keith has, and has already come through the treatment. He is a member of another local Baptist church, and promised prayer for Keith as he completes his treatment. It is so amazing to me how God brings people in and out of our lives at just the time that we need them.

We are looking forward to a quiet weekend, then we go in on Monday for the final treatment....and the ringing of the chemo graduation bell! I'll post a picture on Monday!!!

Monday, November 2

Well, POOH! No chemo graduation bell today! Keith started feeling pretty bad last night, and this morning it was like he had been unplugged. He was really wiped out, and I felt like his counts might be slipping. When they tested him today they found out that both the white count and the hemoglobin were both very low. SO...we had to hold off on the final treatment, and he has to get a transfusion tomorrow. They will test him again on Wednesday, and hopefully will be able to give him the Bleomyicin and ring the chemo bell then!

He is tracking along the same path as he did last round, so I know the transfusion will help. Please pray that the counts will come back up and that he will continue to get stronger and stronger. We are SOOOO ready to be finished with all of this!

Tuesday, November 3

Keith had the transfusion today, and I think it has really helped him. He was so fatigued this morning that he could hardly hold his head up. The doctor ended up ordering platelets for him as well. I am hoping it will really give him a boost.

Last night, he said, "Okay, I'm tired of this. Is there a place that I can say...this is enough?" I told him that I didn't think there was, but we would make it through.

He goes in for bloodwork tomorrow and hopefully the final treatment...so if you hear a bell ringing and lots of cheers from the west coast of Florida...you'll know we are finished!

Wednesday, November 4

Chemo graduation happened today! Hooray! He went in for bloodwork and while the numbers weren't great, they were good enough for him to get hi final treatment. So, at around 2:15 ET, Keith Martin rang the chemo graduation bell, to the cheers of all the nurses in the treatment room!

He did find out today that 3 times in this process he has made "the book" that they keep in the lab for the lowest bloodwork. Apparently when he had the platelet count of 15,000 (remember they sent us straight to the hospital), that was the lowest platelets thay had ever had in the lab there. So, Keith is famous for many things!

They still were not thrilled with his white count, so he has to go back in tomorrow for a neupagin shot. But just to know that he is completely through with the chemo is such a great thing!

Please just be praying now about the scans. We are praying for NO TRACE of the cancer!!

Thursday, November 5

Today has been a little better. The transfusion has helped Keith to feel stronger, but he is really having a hard time eating. The doctor is not sure if that is something related to his lap band or if it has something to do with the chemo. He is going to a different doctor next Tuesday to determine if the lap band needs to be adjusted. He has lost another 3 lbs., so we need to get this part figured out!

He is still planning on leading worship this weekend, and hopefully (if we can get the eating stuff figured out) he will continue to get stronger. The ringing of the chemo bell was such a huge relief...at least now when he does get stronger he won't have to be struck down again by the next round of chemo!

Please pray especially about the eating stuff, that we can get it figured out.

Friday, November 6

Today has been a bit of a challenge. The Neupagin has caused him to have some severe back pain. We have had to pull out the morphine again. As much as we hate to have to do that, it was funny how quickly it helped him. Hopefully by tomorrow the back pain will have subsided. As bad as it is, the pain helps us know that the Neupagin is helping to boost the white count by producing bone marrow. It's quite a circle!

Last night Keith went to the last part of the rehearsal. The choir had already rehearsed, and had come into the Worship Center to do the runthrough with the band. Unbeknownst to Keith, they had pulled out all the bells and chimes from the Children's Choir box and when he came in, the entire choir began ringing bells and chimes to celebrate him ringing the chemo graduation bell! It was great!

Please continue to pray about his eating challenges and about the pain in his back. He is getting stronger, but with every two steps forward, it seems like there is one step back!

Monday, November 9

Keith led worship in our services this past weekend, and did a great job. He got sick during the first service, and wasn't sure he was going to be able to do the last one, but he got to feeling better, so he led the service and Andy stayed around and did the invitation so Keith could go home. He was sick off and on all day yesterday.

This morning he decided to go in to the office for half a day. He got up and put all his stuff in the car, then came in and got sick and had to go back to bed! He was better by lunchtime, and ended up going in this afternoon. He's still having lots of trouble eating. We go in to see the doctor tomorrow to see if his eating issues have anything to do with the lap band. Hopefully I will have more information on that tomorrow afternoon.

Please pray that we will be able to find out the source of the eating problems so he can really begin getting his strength back.

Tuesday, November 10

We went to the doctor today (the lap band doctor), and he felt sure that Keith's eating problems were related to the lap band, so he took out some of the liquid so the band would open up more. For the first time in awhile, Keith was able to eat dinner tonight! And for the first time in an even longer while, we cooked dinner!! It was so nice to grill chicken and fix veggies just like the "old days!" Of course, I am a little spoiled to eating out and take out!!

A week from today will mark the 4 month mark since this journey began. Over those months, Keith has probably received over 300 cards, and 3 times that many emails. He has received so many encouraging words, prayers and well wishes, and we could never tell you how much they have meant to us. Last week, however, we received a letter from a friend that is unlike any of the other cards and letters we have received. It came from a friend of ours, Jennifer Mathewson Speer, who we have known since college days. I have asked her permission to share the letter with you, but before I do, you need to know a little background on her.

As I said, Jennifer became a friend of ours when we were at Samford. She also performed on the team we directed at the World's Fair in 1982. She met her husband, Dana, when we were all at seminary in Ft. Worth, Texas, and we fell in love with him. Dana was a fun-loving, bigger than life pastor who loved his family and God's church. On several occasions Keith contacted Dana to seek his counsel on ministry issues. Life rolled along, and Jennifer and Dana had two children, and lived in Knoxville, Tennessee, where he was a pastor. On the day that we were moving from Indiana to Florida, we got a call in the middle of the night that Dana had been killed in a car accident. He was hit head-on less than a mile from their house, on his way to the church for a meeting.

Since that time, Jennifer has remarried a wonderful man, Alan Speer, who is also a pastor. She lives in a small town in Illinois, and she travels and speaks to women's groups all over the country. I'm trying to talk her into writing a book, and when you read this letter, I think you will agree with me! It is rather lengthy, but I promise you will be richer for having read it.

Keith and Lee Ann,

Throughout my life, people have given me tons of advice. Some of it has been good and some-well, I just listen politely and let it go. But when someone has suffered and decides to speak into my life, I listen intently. You, my friend, have suffered. The Lord, however, will use your suffering to speak into the lives of so many people and they will listen because you have walked a difficult road. I am a fellow member of the "Sufferer's club" so I hope you will indulge me for a few minutes.

I wanted to take a minute and share with you some of the things you might look out for in the months ahead as you continue to walk your journey of both suffering and healing- not just the obstacles that are ahead but the glories that lay just down the way. I also want to warn you about the stupid things people will say and the ridiculous things we as Christians have come to believe.

The most obvious thing that will come from your experience is that you will be more attuned to another's suffering. The apostle Paul was right on when he wrote in 2 Corinthians that we comfort others with the comfort which we ourselves have received. You will understand that every person you meet, whether in Wal-Mart or church, is suffering, has suffered or will suffer on some level.

You will hear more stories of cancer and death, loss and hurt than you ever realized were out there. They have always been there, but you have new ears to hear and understand and a new perspective from which to speak and minister. Speak freely. People want truth. They need to know that cancer sucks, chemo is hell, fear is real, and God is sometimes silent. They will need for you to tell them the good things too: friends matter, prayer helps, family is imperative. Yet in the midst of speaking the truth you will also have to tell them things that we as Christians don't like to grapple with.

It has been four years since Dana was killed and still there are some deep shadows of hurt in my life-especially at church. For four years, I have heard people give testimonies of miraculous healing, divine intervention, deliverance from dangerous situations and even being snatched from the perils of death. In those same testimonies, people will praise the Lord for His protection and declare that their experience is proof that the Lord protects His own. When I hear that, something inside of me aches and grieves all over again and a thousand questions dig into my heart. If God protected them, why not Dana? Why did my boys have to suffer such loss? Why did Dana experience an agonizing nine hour death? Why are we still so wounded? Where was God's protection when death and peril and brokenness attacked us?

*But this is what I have discovered. Even though those testimonies are spoken in good faith, they do not rightly represent God. In this life, we are never, not once, promised the protection of God. We are never told to trust in His protection. (Of course we have eternal protection-our salvation is secure. And there is certainly nothing wrong with asking for protection.) We are, however, always promised the presence of God. The Bible says, "**When** you pass through the waters, **I will be with you**." But if I am trusting primarily in the protection of God, in times of death and sickness and sorrow, my faith will crumble. Instead, I am to trust in God Himself. I am to trust His wisdom and love and sovereignty- the very nature and character of God. In this, I will not be disappointed. Neither will you.*

You will find that in difficult times-even in the aftermath of a difficult journey-some folks will be like Job's friends. They don't mean to be ignorant but they always feel a need to say something. Usually it is the wrong thing. Most of the time they want to help explain why you have been through what you have been through and most of the time they assume God had some great thing to teach you through it all.

I sat with a young widow whose husband of 6 months had been killed in a car accident. She said these profound words to me. "People say that God will teach me so much through all of this. But am I so stupid that this is what God had to use to teach me?" I was speechless. I knew exactly how she felt though I had never verbalized it so plainly.

***The Shack** is one of my favorite books. I know it has been controversial in some circles, but I think you can never fully appreciate it unless you have wrestled with the issue of a good God allowing really bad circumstances into your life. To me, the most eye-opening part of the book is the conversation Mac has with Wisdom. Wisdom tells him that God does not cause or allow bad things to happen SO THAT He can teach us. Bad things happen because we live in a fallen world and in the midst of them*

God reveals Himself to us. So it is not great lessons we are to learn through our pain. It is a great Presence whom we are to experience and trust through our pain. This is true for my young widow friend and for me and for you as well.

You will also find in the years ahead that God redeems the pain. He redeems the pain of feeling rejected by Him. He redeems the pain of loss and sorrow and sickness. Certainly redeem does not mean He makes it all go away. He instead buys it back and refines it into something new. Somehow He makes all the pain coexist with the joy of His presence and His grace. He reshapes the brokenness into His image-and you will shine differently than ever before.

A benefit of difficult circumstances is the way you will live from day to day. You will never leave relationships unresolved or broken. Life is too short and too precious. You will love deeper, grieve harder, laugh louder, hold tighter. The unimportant things of life will become glaringly unimportant. You will never walk out of the house or go on a trip that you do not take Lee Ann in your arms and confirm your love for her a thousand times. If you let it, sickness and loss and tragedy will make your marriage more passionate than it has ever been.

Finally, be careful around ungrateful people-especially church folks. You will find that you are more impatient and less tolerant of people who whine and complain-you know the type. The kind of person that gripes because the building is too hot or cold; or they didn't get the solo, or their child was overlooked, or their feelings got hurt, or the sermon was too long and the music too loud. You will want to scream at them, "Try having cancer!" Restrain yourself. They won't ever get it. At least not until God blesses them with something really worth complaining about.

In the end, you are different. I have cried many times for the privilege of having my life back the way it was before death and suffering invaded. But it won't ever be the same. Consequently, I now know that anything can happen to anybody. I always knew that in my head but because I had never experienced something so personally horrible, I could not know that truth completely. In light of this knowledge, there is a tendency to always be waiting for the next bad thing to happen to you or to those you love; waiting for the next proverbial shoe to fall. There will be the tendency to let fear rule. Don't let it. It is destructive and will lead you into terrible bondage. I know that from experience. Yes, something terrible might happen again in the future, but the Lord has been with you in the past and will give grace to face whatever comes in the future. Live in His presence one moment at a time.

You are my dear friend. You and Lee Ann have been a constant source of love and leadership for me. You both have been woven throughout every season of my life for the last 32 years and I am deeply thankful for the blessings you have added each step of the way.

You have been given a difficult but profound experience. Your cancer certainly will not define you but oh how it will define Christ in you. I love you both.

Jennifer

Thursday, November 12

Okay...no morbid stories or gut wrenching letters tonight...just good news! Keith went to the office for a full day today! He went to staff meeting for the first time since June. Then he stayed all day and into rehearsals tonight. I haven't seen him yet, but I'm sure he will be one tired boy when he gets in!

So now our attention turns to the scan on Monday. My stomach turns a little when I think about it, as it will determine the "what's next" in our lives. We are praying that the cancer will be gone...nothing to take out...nothing to "watch." But, as you know from walking this journey with us, we will travel whatever path God has for us.

Friday, November 13

As predicted, Keith was wiped out when he got in last night. He had been at the office all day, went straight into Praise Team rehearsal, then choir rehearsal, then the weekend run-through, then stayed after to hear someone sing. Oh, and in between work and Praise Team he met with the Physical Therapist that is helping him with his muscle weakness.

SO, today was a lazy day. He slept late, then we went to lunch, and both came back and took a nap! He was so wiped out this morning. Hopefully it has made him realize that he has to work up to days like that.

We hit out first insurance snag since this whole ordeal has started today. The radiologist called to say that our insurance had declined the PET scan that was scheduled for Monday. They have approved the CT scan, but would not approve the PET with Keith's particular type of cancer. I drew my guns, ready to take on the insurance company, but I talked with the doctor's office financial lady, and she said that Dr. Berry would see if the CT showed him everything he needed to see, or if we needed to take on the insurance company for the PET. She said if we had to challenge the insurance that it would take about a month for them to review the claim and determine to pay for the test. She said the felt sure they would approve it if Dr. Berry went to bat for it, but it would just take time. Apparently it is a VERY expensive test.

So, please pray this weekend that the CT scan will be clear and will give the doctor all the answers he needs. I trust this doctor, and if he has any questions he will fight to get the answers. It's just in "Keith and Lee Ann world" we are ready to be done with all of this!

Monday, November 16

Well, Keith had the scan today. Everything went fine, and we went down to the beach and ate lunch at one of his favorite restaurants. We ate right out on the sand. It was a gorgeous day, and was so nice to be there together again.

Now we just have to hurry up and wait again. We should get the results when we meet with the doctor at 1:15 on Thursday. I'm really praying that he will say something like, "Hmmmm...what cancer? We can't seem to find any!!"

If you haven't taken a minute to watch the video above, please do. Although Keith is weak, you can tell he has a renewed passion. Our friend, Paul Strozier, from Ohio had the following comment:

"I watched the video on the website and wanted you to know that I got saved again! I even took a little offering from myself right here in my office. It just seemed appropriate.

I knew you would be even more sensitive and that the Holy Spirit's power and anointing would be even more evident in your ministry as you went on this journey, but I couldn't imagine how powerful it would be. God is loving you and using you my friend. Don't stop! It is the power of God to save lives!"

Keith has bloodwork tomorrow and then the appointment on Thursday. Thank you for your prayers. I think we are both a little nervous about getting the results.

Tuesday, November 17

I am writing early today, as many of you have already heard the events of yesterday afternoon. I should have updated this last night, but I was just beat by the time we got back home. Okay, I'm getting ahead of myself. Let me back up to yesterday afternoon.

Keith finished the scan yesterday around 2 pm. We went to lunch and got home around 3. He went to the office and I sat down to do some more work. Around 4 pm the phone rang, and it was one of the nurses from the Cancer Center. She said, "We need for Mr. Martin to come back down here today or no later than tomorrow morning." Of course, this was the SAME phone call we got from the doctor back on July 17 after that scan, so my thoughts immediately went to another mass or something worse.

I knew that Keith was in a meeting with Tim, our pastor, so I said, " I don't think we can be there before you close today, but we can come first thing in the morning." And then I said, "but I need to know why we are coming, or we won't sleep a wink tonight." She left to speak to Keith's nurse and came back and said, "He has a blood clot in his lung." To which I responded..."We'll be right there!"

I called Keith and he dropped everything and we made it down there in record time. Turns out he has a small Pulmonary Embolism (blood clot) in his lung. The very great news is that the only reason they found it was because of the scan. The nurse told him that God really had His hand on Keith, as most of these clots are not discovered until they get big enough to start producing symptoms.

They gave him a Heparin shot yesterday and he will get one of those every day this week. He has also started on Coumidin (blood thinner) to keep the clot from getting larger or new clots forming. They said this is caused by the chemotherapy, and they see it in the office at least once a week, but it was sure scary to us!

When we finally got back home and collapsed on the couch yesterday evening, Keith joked, "Well, I could tell I wasn't the center of the universe any more, so I had to do something to get things back as they needed to be!"

And, I'm sure you are wondering, "what about the tumor?" We don't know anything yet, and will not know until we meet with the doctor on Thursday. No one that we met with yesterday had seen that part of the results. I think the clot trumped everything!

So, a new thing to add to the prayer list...blood clot. Please pray that it stays small and the medicines enable Keith's body to reabsorb it. Also, please be thankful that they found this so early.

What a journey!

Wednesday, November 18

Believe it or not, today has been rather uneventful on the healthcare front. Of course, it's only 5 pm, so there's still plenty of time for action!! Keith went in to get the Heparin shot today, and whatever it is they are trying to do had gone down instead of up. The are trying to get his blood to a 2, and right now he is at a 1.1. He has to keep getting the Heparin until it reaches the magic number. So, please pray with us about that.

We have the appointment with the doctor tomorrow morning at 9 am. That's when we will hear the results of the scan, and what is next for us. We go from there into staff meeting at church, but I promise to write as soon as I get home and let you know the results. We are both a little nervous, but ready to see what is going on inside of him (besides blood clots!)

Thursday, November 19

Okay, we finally have the results of the scan! The news is very good, but not great. "Great" to us would have been that the cancer was completely gone! That's not the case. The mass has, however, shrunk substantially again. It is now 2" x 2". The doctor is very pleased with that. The next step is to get the insurance to approve the PET scan, because we have to find out if there is any residual cancer in the mass. If there is, then he will have to go to Moffitt in Tampa to have it surgically removed. If there is not, then he will have scans for every 6 months for 2 years to be sure there is no change, then they will declare him "cured." (quoting the doctor) He said that over the next few years that the remaining tumor would be absorbed by the body if no cancer cells remained.

SO...the URGENT prayer request is that the insurance will approve the test. Doctor Berry wants it done as soon as possible, because he said that if there is residual cancer, there is a chance that it could start growing again, and nobody wants that. Our insurance has said that it may take 30-45 days for the approval process to happen. I am going to call them this afternoon, and the Cancer Center is also doing the formal request from the doctor, so please just pray that they will approve the test quickly.

They have scheduled for Keith to have an ultrasound of his legs this afternoon to check for more clots. The doctor actually suspects that he does have more clots, but doesn't seem real concerned about it! Keith is still taking the Heparin, and his INR is at 1.3 today (we need it at 2).

The picture I had in my mind of Keith and I skipping happily into the sunset with this behind us is not a reality yet, but we have sure come a long way down the road. And I say with all sincerity that we could not have reached this point without all of you and your support and prayers.

Update:
I just had a call from Keith and the test showed that his legs are clear...no clots! Praise God!

Friday, November 20

Writing a little late tonight, but it is because we have been at Disney today! We went with our "Metro" friends, the Moores and the Cranes, and Greg pushed Keith around in a wheelchair! It was such a great day...the weather was beautiful, and it was great to just be doing something fun!

I posted a brief message yesterday afternoon that Keith's legs were clear of any clots. We are so glad of that! His INR today is at 1.6, so he will have to go to the hospital tomorrow and Sunday to get the Heparin shot.

I also have some insurance news. Our doctor's office called the insurance company yesterday and was very persistent that the 30-45 day period to determine if the scan would be approved was not acceptable, especially since it put Keith's health in jeopardy. She managed to speak with somebody high up enough that told her that the case would be marked as a priority, and they would have and answer on it by Tuesday. So, our doctor has set up the scan for Wednesday morning, anticipating that it will be approved on Tuesday. Please pray with us that they will approve it so he can have the scan on Wednesday and we can know whether or not the cancer cells are still there. And, of course we are praying that they find no cancer!

Monday, November 23

Keith went to the hospital for Heparin shots over the weekend, and today his INR was at 3.1. That's great news, and means he doesn't have to have any more shots!

Bethany came in on Saturday, and my mom and Josh both arrived today. We are looking forward to a great family week! The last time Josh was here was back in July when Keith was in the hospital, so needless to say, Keith looks a little different since then! Mom had not seen Keith since May! They had both seen photos, but they don't quite do him justice!

We should find out tomorrow about the insurance approval of the PET scan. It is scheduled for Wednesday morning at 8:30 am, so hopefully all will be approved. Please pray with us about that. I'll let you know tomorrow as soon as we know something.

Tuesday, November 24

Well, good news, finally...late this afternoon the insurance approved the PET scan. Our doctor had to actually speak with one of the insurance doctors. He did, and the scan was approved for 3 weeks after Keith finished treatment. That would actually be this week, but our doctor wants us to wait until December 9. The interesting thing is that the scan had actually been denied a second time, but when they did the peer to peer conference, our doctor was able to convince them of the necessity. I am so thankful for a doctor who is willing to go the extra mile!

Our doctor is referring us to Moffitt Cancer Center for evaluation. I'm not really sure why, but it's been too long of a day to worry about that today. According to his nurse, he wants to have everything ready in case Keith has to have surgery after the PET. Like I said, we'll think about that next week!

So...as has been our theme through this journey....hurry up and wait!

Wednesday, November 25

Moffitt Cancer Center called today to set up the consult for Keith. He is going to be with a Dr. Sexton, who is supposedly a highly respected doctor there. The appointment is scheduled for January 8, but the nurse said that if our doctor wanted him to see Dr. Sexton earlier, he just needed to contact them and they would work Keith in.

No one has told us for sure, but we assume that if the PET scan on the 9th shows that there is cancer still in the mass, they will bump up the Moffitt appointment to make a surgery decision. If there is no cancer, we assume that our doctor wants this doctor to look at Keith's case to be sure they still do not want to surgically remove what's left. Either way, Moffitt is such a respected hospital, and it is good to know that they are going to look over Keith's case.

It is great to have everyone here. We have laughed and talked and laughed some more. It's all good medicine for Keith!

Thursday, November 26 - Thanksgiving Day

Today we are thankful for...friends; family; a network of prayer warriors; a great doctor; adequate health insurance; the person who years ago discovered the treatment for testicular cancer; but most of all for a relationship with a God who walks with us through whatever we face.

Happy Thanksgiving

Friday, November 27

This has been a wonderful holiday! Having our family here has been great. Mom and Josh both head back tomorrow. Bethany went back yesterday, as she had tickets to the Alabama-Auburn game. She was really holding out hope for a great upset today, but , of course, Keith was greatly relieved that Alabama pulled it out!

It has been so nice to pull away and just enjoy family and not think about doctors and illness. I know it will all still be there on Monday, but I'll think about it then!!

Monday, November 30

We had such a wonderful time visiting with our family this past week. The last time Josh was here was when Keith was in the hospital in July. Bethany has been in since then, but Josh has only kept in touch via phone. My mom hasn't seen Keith since last May! Needless to say, he could have walked by her on the street and she would not have known him!

We had a lot of fun and interesting talks remembering this journey. It's really funny all of the things Keith doesn't remember at the beginning when he was on morphine. He doesn't even remember getting a brain scan! I think that would haunt me for life! And there are MANY conversations and visits that he doesn't remember. We have had a lot of laughs reminding him of some of the crazy things he said and did when he was on morphine and Ambien!

He goes in tomorrow for blood work and to get more information on the PET scan. As far as we know, it is scheduled for Wednesday, December 9. The insurance approved it for 3 weeks after he completed treatment. It is scheduled now for 3 weeks after the CT scan, which may be what signals the end of treatment. Whatever the case, we are just very pleased that it is back on the docket!

Tuesday, December 1

Keith went to the Cancer Center today for bloodwork. His counts were pretty good...red count is inching up, but white count is a little lower. His INR (for the blood thinning) has come down, so they are altering his medicine again to try and get it back up to a 2.

Several of you have asked why we are waiting until December 9 for the PET scan since the insurance approved it. Come to find out, the insurance approved it for 6 weeks after Keith finished treatment. That was totally unacceptable to our doctor, so they are fussing about that with the insurance company. I think he forgot, however, that Keith's final treatment was November 4, and the scan is scheduled for December 9, which is 5 weeks. So, I guess worse case scenerio is that we will have to wait until the 16th or 17th to have it done which will be the full 6 weeks. We are just SO READY to have it done so we can know what the next step is!!

Wednesday, December 2

BIG NEWS....Keith had to shave today!! First time since August! We went out to dinner last night, and I looked over at him and said, "You are beginning to look scruffy!" He had little gray peach fuzz all over his face. It's a little thing, but it is a step back toward normalcy. Not that he really missed shaving, but it is nice to feel like his body is coming back to normal!

We had meetings all morning, and Keith has rehearsals all evening, so he came home and rested this afternoon. He has found that if he goes nonstop all day on rehearsal days it will affect him for a couple of days afterward. He's sort of learning what he can do and what he can't. He's so much stronger than he was just a few weeks ago, and every day is getting a little stronger!

Thursday, December 3

Keith has been really dealing with the fatigue today. I think it may be partially due to the change in the Coumidin medication. Tonight he said, "I really wonder if I am ever going to feel normal again. And today I really felt like the answer to that is no." Of course I tried to assure him that he will be normal again, and I really believe that he will, but it is so difficult to see him so down. He just needs a boost of energy!

Please pray that he will continue to gain his strength back, and that all will move forward with the PET scan. I think the pressure of not knowing whether or not there will be more to the story is really weighing on him.

Friday, December 4

Today was a good day. We did some Christmas shopping, and went out to dinner. It was rainy and dark here all day, which is about as close to a "snow day" as we get here in Florida. It really is rare to have a day where it rains all day! So tonight it was nice to hear the rain outside and cuddle up by the Christmas tree. And...just for the record...been there and done that on the snow - and we DON'T miss it! I'll take rain and 65 degrees any time!

The cancer center called today to be sure that Keith has heard from Moffitt. She said they are still planning on the PET scan next Wednesday, but they are still haggling with the insurance. We think that the worse case scenerio is that the test will be on the 17th. That is 6 weeks after he finished treatment. We are just ready to have it!

Monday, December 7

What a great weekend we had! Our services were great, and Alabama triumphed in the SEC Championship! To all of you Florida fans that love Keith Martin, please take consolation in the fact that Alabama football this year has really been a bright spot in a very difficult Fall! Okay, maybe that's no consolation, but he sure was happy!

We are still in the "hurry up and wait" mode regarding the PET scan, but for now it is scheduled for Wednesday. We should find out tomorrow afternoon if it is really going to happen. Keith got the information packet from Moffitt Cancer Center over the weekend, and it is very impressive. They have an entire department devoted to the treatment of bladder, testicular, and prostate cancer. It's called the "Genitourinary Oncology Program." I had to look that word up online to be sure Keith didn't have some new disease!!

So, please pray that we can get the scan and move forward to whatever is next!

Tuesday, December 8

Hooray, Hooray, and three times Hooray! We found out today that all is on for the PET scan tomorrow. The insurance has approved it, and Keith is all set for it at 10:30 am. I'm not sure when we will find out any results, but I know it will be at least a couple of days, and it will probably be next week. I promise as soon as we know something that I will put it here.

Keith had his bloodwork done today and it wasn't great. His red count is still low, and the INR was at 1.5. So, more Coumidin! It's a good thing it's 75 degrees here in Florida...he wouldn't survive in a colder climate. If it get's down to 60, he thinks he's dying!!

Please pray for him as he has the test tomorrow. We REALLY are praying for accurate results so that there will be no doubt as to what needs to happen next. Of course we are asking that there be no cancer remaining!

Wednesday, December 9

Keith had the scan today. All went well, except they told him for the rest of the day to stay away from small children or pregnant women since he would still have radioactivity in his body. That was pretty creepy! We don't anticipate hearing any results until next week. So...again...hurry up and wait!

Yesterday Keith had someone introduce him as a "cancer survivor." That was a first, and while I guess he is a survivor because he's still breathing, we still don't feel like this is behind us yet . Maybe when the doctor says, "Okay, there's no more cancer, go and live your life!" But, even if those words are never spoken, he is a survivor, and we are so thankful for it.

Our life is in high gear right now getting ready for our Christmas program this weekend. Several of you have asked, and it will be broadcast online through our live streaming. The times are Saturday at 5 pm, and Sunday at 9 and 10:45 am (ET). Keith is going to speak about his journey. I know it will be great. If you think about it, please join us online. If you are close enough to come, then join us in person!

Thursday, December 10

Okay, so we have a LITTLE bit of news. When we got in from rehearsal tonight (at 10:30 pm) we had a message from our doctor that he had the results of the scan and felt good about it. He wanted Keith to call him, but obviously we weren't going to call him at 10:30! He said he still wants Keith to keep the appointment at Moffitt, but he said he was very encouraged by the results. So, what that means is anybody's guess! I'm sure Keith will try and contact him tomorrow, so we'll let you know if we find out anything!

Rehearsal for our Christmas program went well tonight. It's really a pretty good program considering the Worship Pastor has had cancer for the past 5 months!

Friday, December 11

We are back in the waiting room again....Keith Helped with a funeral this morning and by the time he got home and could call the Cancer Center they had closed for the day. They don't normally close at noon on Friday, but today they did. SO....we will have to wait until Monday to kow the final results of the scan. I keep hearing the doctor say, "I am very encouraged by what I see on the scan." And if he's encouraged, we are encouraged! I promise to let you know if we find out anything.

This cooler weather we are having here is about to wipe Keith out! We went to dinner tonight, and the temp is around 60 degrees. I wore jeans and a t-shirt. Keith had on a polo shirt, a sweatshirt, a coat and a wool cap!! Just imagine if he lived where some of you do and the temp was around 17!!

If you can, join us in person or online (www.woodlandlive.com) this weekend to see our Christmas program. Services are Saturday at 5 pm and Sunday at 9 and 10:45 am.

Monday, December 14

Keith talked to the doctor today, and here's what we know...the scan showed that the tumor had shrunk even more since the CT scan. It is now 1.6 x 1.9 inches. The scan showed that the material is "inactive" which we think means no cancer, but Keith didn't actually ask that question! The spot by his shoulder blade is gone, and the spots in his groin area are gone (he had one by his liver and one by his kidney). He was concerned about something that he saw in Keith's lung...don't worry, not cancer, but an irritation that the chemo had caused. He said he wanted Keith to be aware of his breathing and if he seemed short of breath, he wanted to know that at his appt. on Thursday and he might send him to a lung doctor. All in all, we are praising the Lord for this report! We just can't hardly let ourselves believe that the cancer might actually be gone!!

Our program this weekend went great, but Keith was one tired puppy when we got home. We are out the door right now to head over to Orlando for a couple of days at Disney. We are meeting friends tonight for the Candlelight Processional, and then Bethany is coming in tonight and will spend the day with us there tomorrow. She is finishing finals today. Don't worry, we are Disney season pass holders, so we don't do Disney like the average tourist. We take it slow....!

Because we will be gone, I will not be writing tomorrow (first weekday I will have missed since July!) I'll be back again on Wednesday. Please be praying about this lung thing. I am really hoping it is nothing!

Wednesday, December 16

We had a great few days at Disney. The Candlelight Processional was fabulous! Scripture and music celebrating the birth of Christ...right in the middle of Disney! Bethany got there late Monday night and we had a great day yesterday with her. She and Keith squared off for Toy Story Mania, and she almost beat him!

When we got home we had a message from the doctors office that they had his bloodwork back and his potassium is low. the nurse told him to eat bananas and drink Gatorade to try and build it up. It's always something!

We see the doctor tomorrow morning and I think we will have a clearer picture after we talk to him. I'll post as soon as I get home tomorrow to let you know what we find out. Hopefully what we inferred from the phone conversation is true, and there is no cancer remaining!

Thursday, December 17

We heard the words today that we have been waiting to hear for a long time. Keith was diagnosed with cancer on July 17, and today, December 17, 5 months later, we heard the doctor say, "You are CANCER FREE!!" Followed in my head by a brief rendition of the Hallelujah Chorus and me saying to myself, "Don't cry...don't cry!"

He is considered to be in remission, and they will have to watch him for 3 years or so. If it doesn't come back by then, they will consider him cured. The doctor said it has a 10-20% chance of returning, as there may be some rogue cancer cells that were not terminated. He said that's why they gave Keith the 4th treatment, to "mop up" (his words) any remaining cancer cells in the blood stream or in the mass.

So...now the challenge is to help his body recover from all that they did to him while making him cancer free! He has an inflammation in his lung from the Bleomyicin, and is having trouble with his legs from the Cisplatin. His blood counts are slowly moving up, but now his Potassium is low. His hair is starting to grow back (I told him today that he looked like a Chia Pet...he was not amused!) and he actually had a 5 o'clock shadow last night (of course it takes him 3 days to get it!).

We have an appointment with the lung doctor next week, and the doctor still wants us to keep the appointment with the doctor at Moffitt in January. He does not anticipate that the doctor is going to want to remove the remaining mass, but he wants the surgeon to make the final decision.

So hard to believe this day has finally arrived, and we absolutely could not have travelled this path without you, your support, and your prayers. We are so blessed to call you friends.

Friday, December 18

Today has been filled with preparation for a reception tonight honoring our technical director, who will be leaving us at the end of the year. While it was a busy day, Keith was unusually tired, To the point that I called the cancer center just to be sure it wasn't something we needed to be concerned about. They have started him on Prednisone for the lung inflammation, and I was afraid it might have something to do with that. The nurse said it didn't, and probably the events of the past week and weekend were just catching up with him. He rested the remainder of the day, and did fine at the party tonight.

This week Keith has tried to make a point to honor and thank his staff for the work they did this year. They went above and beyond by stepping in July-October to keep the program running. Our people were so faithful, too. The choir grew and there was anticipation and excitement about Keith's return. So when he did come back, he was able to step right in , not rebuild a program that had been on hold for 4 months. We are so thankful for that.

We talked at lunch today that we will probably finish out the blog next week. He wants to write something for me to post, and we still have to compile the list of the "Top 10 Good Things About Chemo." How appropriate that we finish things up on Christmas week!

Monday, December 21

We went to see the lung doctor today. Keith is definitely short of breath, and has trouble breathing even when leading in worship. The doctor looked over the CT Scan and the PET Scan and said that he really didn't see anything that would be causing the problem. He did a chest x ray on Keith and said that while his lungs did not look quite normal, they did not look bad enough to be causing breathing problems.

So, he wants Keith to have another Muga scan to check on the functionality of his heart, as the Bleomyicin can weaken the heart muscle. He is supposed to have that done tomorrow or Wednesday. We are really praying it is normal, because the doctor told us that if his heart has been affected, that is usually not reversable.

It could also be that he is just exhausted from trying too soon to get back into his routine. But hey...you try and tell him to slow down! I'll let you know what we find out from the Muga.

Tuesday, December 22

Today was a good day of winding up work projects and doing Christmas odds and ends. Keith worked all day, planning and scheduling for next year. He really likes working during this week, because no one is in the office!

His breathing is a lot better today. I am really starting to wonder if he has just worn himself out trying to get back into his routine too fast. The week before the Christmas program he worked 12 hour days, and then did the dress rehearsal and 3 services over the weekend. Hopefully that is it and he will just keep getting stronger.

The Muga scan is scheduled for 10 am tomorrow. Please pray that his heart muscle is normal. We meet with the cancer doctor on Christmas Eve, and should have the results then.

Keith's hair is starting to come back a little. It is still very short, but it is trying. I think he is going to let it grow and see what it looks like, then make the decision if he wants to shave it again. this morning, for fun, he reached into his drawer in the bathroom, pulled out his brush and acted like he was brushing it! Not quite enough there yet for brushing!!

Wednesday, December 23

Josh came in tonight, so now we have the whole family here! It is so good to just relax and visit, especially against the backdrop of the year that we have had. Keith had the Muga scan today, and we should know the results of it tomorrow. We have an appointment with the cancer doctor in the morning, yes, on Christmas Eve!!

Okay, as promised, here is our version of

The Top 10 Good Things About Chemo

1. Experiencing the overwhelming love of a wonderful church and staff at Woodland, as well as the many hundreds of friends who have contacted us and prayed for us through this journey. We can never express the gratitude that is in our hearts for you.
2. Receiving over 300 cards and notes .
3. LOTS of time to reflect on life (over 100 hours in the chemo chair!)
4. People come in from out of town to clean your house and organize your garage (thanks, Paul & Mariann!)
5. You have the chance to look like Tim Passmore!
6. You never have to miss a game when Alabama plays at 3:30 on Saturday!
7. When there is a staff workday, you don't have to participate!
8. No shaving for eight weeks!
9. You save lots of money on hair products and haircuts, and you NEVER have to worry about whether or not your hair looks okay!
10. Losing 45 pounds! Okay, the diet is not recommended, but the results are great!

But the most important "Good thing" about the journey that we have been on is knowing day by day, hour by hour, that God was walking every step with us. We were amazed by the number of times that He had gone before us to prepare the way. Whatever the future holds, we know that we know that we KNOW that God is real and loves us so much.

When I sent out the first email to our friends back in July about Keith, I wrote the following, "For over 30 years we have been telling people that God is trustworthy. Now it is is time to trust." I am here now to tell you that He IS trustworthy! Amen and Amen.

Monday, December 28

Sorry I didn't report back after our visit with the cancer doctor, and thank you to those of you that emailed, concerned about the results. The reason I didn't was because we really didn't find out anything. Dr. Berry didn't have any results on the Muga scan, but he really feels like Keith's heart is fine. He thinks the lung problems are probably just a result of the drugs, and will get better with time. Keith is doing SO much better in all areas. His strength is better, his breathing is better, and his hair and eyebrows are starting to grow back. I think he may shave his head again, since the hair that is coming is sort of scruffy and gray, but this time on HIS terms!

We had a wonderful Christmas! Josh and Bethany were both here, as well as my mom. It is amazing after you go through the year that we have experienced, those family times become even more special.

Keith has bloodwork tomorrow, and hopefully his red count will come up some. It is still low. He doesn't see the doctor again until next week, but hopefully we will find out something about the test today.

Tuesday, December 29

Keith went to the doctor today for bloodwork, and his INR is at 2.4. That's really good, so they are adjusting the Coumidin accordingly. He's feeling better and stronger every day, and for that we are so grateful.

He had me shave his head again today. He was letting the hair grow back in, but it was growing back gray and scruffy, so he wanted me to go ahead and have it. I think Bethany influenced him, as well, as she told him she really liked it better shaved. His eyebrows are coming back, and that helps so much in him looking less like a cancer patient. His color is good, his eyebrows are bushy (okay, we are on our way to bushy!) and he's even thinking about a little beard of some kind....the new Keith emerges!!

Monday, January 4

Just when I think we are finished, something new comes along. He went back to the lung doctor today for a routine follow up after he had the Muga scan. The scan showed his heart function is fine, but the doctor was still concerned about Keith's shortness of breath. He took a chest xray and saw some things that concerned him. Again, the concern is not that this is cancer, but that it is some sort of inflammation or scar tissue caused by the chemo drugs. SO...we have another CT scan scheduled for tomorrow. This one is a non contrast just for his lungs.

We are in the process of gathering up all the scans and biopsies to take with us to Moffitt on Friday. He's had so many done, it's wonder he doesn't glow when the lights are out! I'm looking forward to meeting this doctor. Friday will just be a consultation, then he will review all of Keith's scans and let us know his recommendation as far as surgery.

Bethany is still home, and this morning woke up with a 103 fever! I took her to the doctor and they said she has strep. So now whe's on an antibiotic, and is bound and determined to head back to Auburn on Wednesday.

Please pray about Keith's lung situation, and especially that they can tell from the scan what we are dealing with.

Tuesday, January 5

Keith had the scan done today. Boy, what a difference the new year makes...suddenly our deductibles and coinsurance are back in the picture! I was sort of used to that 100% coverage that we had from July on last year! Something tells me at the rate we are going, we will hit that $3000 out of pocket pretty soon!

Several of you have asked whether the doctor thinks the lung problems are permanent. At the last visit he told us that the lung issues should get better with time, but if there was a weakness in his heart muscle, then that would be permanent. That's why we were very relieved that the Muga scan came out okay. Of course, I think they have to actually figure out what;s wrong with the lung before they can make a judgment about how to treat it.

Bethany is doing better today. She is planning on traveling back to Auburn tomorrow, ahead of a potential snowstorm scheduled for Thursday there.

Wednesday, January 6

Not much news today. This is the only day this week that Keith hasn't had to go to the doctor. He goes back to the lung doctor tomorrow for review of the lung CT scan, and then to Moffitt on Friday. As soon as we know something about the scan I will post it tomorrow. His appointment is not until 4 pm, so it will be late afternoon.

Bethany left to go back to Auburn today, so it is once again just Keith and I in the house. First time since December 19! We miss her, but she was anxious to get back to school. There is potential for snow tomorrow in Auburn!!

Thursday, January 7

Keith saw the lung specialist today, and the CT scan showed that he has a great deal of inflammation in his lungs. The doctor said that it could be one of 3 things : 1. cancer, which he doesn't suspect, since Keith has just finished chemo, and the PET scan did not show anything there; 2. infection, but he doesn't think it is that, since Keith is not sick; or 3. inflammation or scar tissue, which is most likely what it is, and can be caused by the Bleomyicin. He has put Keith back on Prednizone and wants to check him again in 2 weeks. The good news is that if it is inflammation, the Prednizone should take care of it.

We go to Moffitt tomorrow and plan on asking the doctor there about the lung thing. We have all of the scans and biopsies packed up and ready to go. I'm really looking forward to this next step. Moffitt is such a highly respected cacer center, and I'm glad they will be reviewing Keith's case.

Friday, January 8

Wow...the trip to Moffitt today was unbelievable! It was wonderful, yet overwhelming! First of all, the facility is very impressive. I didn't realize that people come from all over the world to this cancer hospital. It runs like a well-oiled machine! We were there for 3 HOURS...yet we went from step to step before we finally met with the doctor. Come to find out, this doctor is very highly respected and an expert in the area of testicular cancer. He took the time today to review all of Keith's tests and scans, and came into our appointment with a knowledge of Keith's case.

To summarize the 3 HOUR appointment...he showed us the CT scan of the tumor and where it is located. He is not totally convinced that there is no cancer remaining in the tumor. He doesn't suspect that there is, but he can't say with certainty that the cancer is gone. He is going to take Keith's case to the "tumor board" on Monday for review. They will look at all of the factors (tumor location, PET scans, etc.) and make a recommendation as to whether or not the tumor should be removed.

If we decide to have the tumor removed, it is a major surgery...I'm talking Big Boy Surgery, where he would be cut from under his breastbone to just below his navel. The doctor told him that it would be a bit challenging to get to the location of the tumor. Keith said, "You know it's serious surgery when the doctor says he's going to pull out your bowels and lay them aside in order to get to the tumor!!" The recovery time would be about six weeks. The problem with the surgery is that the tumor is still attached to the Veina Cava (sp) and kidney veins, and it is very close to his aorta. The doctor says, however, that they do this surgery all the time.

If they decide not to recommend the surgery, we would just watch the tumor, and would do scans and check it about every three months. The concern is that since the cancer has already moved through Keith's bloodstream that it could happen again if there is any cancer left in the tumor.

So, it is really a Catch 22 situation...the surgery would eradicate the tumor and hopefully any cancer, but it is radical surgery. The waiting and watching holds a risk for the cancer to come back, and plus the tumor is still taking up a good amount of space in his abdomen and pressing on some of his veins.

Needless to say, we were so overwhelmed with all of this information that when we got home we just crashed! It was rainy and cold here, so we came home and took a nap. I think that also had something to do with staying up til 1 am for the Alabama game! Roll tide! We have had a chance to talk about it all a little this evening, which has been good.

The good news is that we feel wonderfully confident with this doctor, and blessed to be within driving distance of a cancer center like this. We really need you all to pray for this tumor board and their decision on Monday. Please ask God to guide them as they are making the decision and recommendation that could affect the rest of Keith's life. We will have information on this on Tuesday, and if they schedule the surgery, it would probably be in a couple of months,

Thank you for your prayers....we will keep you posted!

Saturday, January 9

I am adding a note to my post from last night. We found out after I had written last night that our dear friend, Jackie Decker, lost her fight with cancer yesterday. Jackie is the wife of one of our staff members at Woodland. She and Keith took several chemo treatments together at the cancer center, and I was always amazed at how she sought to minister to those around her, even when she was really feeling rough. Her happy smile and excited greetings when she saw you were genuine and blessed.

This is especially piercing given the journey that we have been on. Please pray for Mike and their children as they go through this. He has been a strong helpmate and caregiver throughout her fight that began last May.

I really hate this insidious disease, but I believe with all my heart that God knows each of our lifespans, and has a plan for each day. Jackie fulfilled that plan, even when hit with some pretty horrifying circumstances. I think today she is being rewarded for that.

Monday, January 11

Well...the plot thickens!! Not really, but it is interesting to compare doctor's appointments. We met with our oncologist today and his opinion is that the PET scan is accurate and there is no more cancer. He said that a surgeon will always be biased toward surgery, because then you know for sure that it is gone and there are no more concerns. He seemed quite concerned with the location of the tumor, and he thinks the tumor board will be, too.

He and I decided (Keith just listened...he didn't agree or disagree!) that the best course of action may be the one that will automatically happen because of Keith's lungs. Our doctor thinks that they will not do the surgery until they can get Keith's lungs back where they need to be. That will probably take several months. What I would like is for us to be able to hold off on the surgery for several months, and then do a scan again before we do it. Dr. Berry said that the tumor is still shrinking, and there is no evidence of cancer, so there is no reason to rush the surgery. That is my gut feeling, too. (And during those months we can have all of you guys praying that the tumor shrinks to nothing and no surgery is needed!!)

Of course, everything may change tomorrow when we hear the recommendation of the tumor board. This is always interesting...I'm just so glad Keith is feeling better and stronger. We'll tackle whatever is ahead!

Tuesday, January 12

We are in Auburn, Alabama today, here to celebrate Bethany's 20th birthday tomorrow. It was a high value to Keith, after the events of the past year, that we be with both of our kids on their birthdays this year. Southwest helped with low fares, so we are doing a bit of a whirlwind trip.

In the midst of our travel today, Keith had a message from the Moffitt doctor. He said that the tumor board had first of all determined that the inflammation in Keith's lungs is from the chemo, and is not cancer. He said that they feel like they are going to "do something with him" as far as surgery, but they want to use the time that his lungs are healing to do more tests. There is a Moffitt lady that is supposed to call to schedule what sounds like a large battery of tests. SO...pretty much sounds like that the tumor board agreed with me :-) ....let's wait and let Keith get stronger and then make the decision about surgery. The only difference is that they are pretty convinced that the surgery will be happening at some point in the future, whereas I'm claiming that when we get to that point, the tumor will have shrunk down to nothing! I am certainly not opposed to the surgery, I just want to be sure Keith is strong enough for it.

So, bottom line is that the tumor board seemed to recommend surgery, but only after Keith's lungs have healed. I'm not really sure what all the new tests are for, but I figure more information can be nothing but good. Keith is going to try and contact them tomorrow, so I'll let you know if we know any more.

Thursday, January 14

Our celebration of Bethany's birthday was wonderful! We had a great day yesterday, and even had a glass of lemonade at Toomer's Corner! For those who don't know, that's quite an Auburn tradition!

Today was a day of traveling, and we had rehearsals tonight. The only news that I have from the cancer front is that we had a message from Moffitt saying that Keith has a MRI scheduled at Moffitt on Friday, Jan 22. I am hoping he can actually talk to the doctor tomorrow and find out a little clearer picture as to what he is planning.

I enjoyed the comments that we got from several of you regarding my assessment that the Moffitt Tumor board agreed with me. This was my favorite, from our friend, Paul Strozier, "OK – I'm thinking we could have just told the Tumor Board that LeeAnn is the Holy Spirit and saved them some meeting time. You could just go ahead and diagnose everything else and save that battery of tests, you know!" That sounds good to me!! I'm glad people are finally starting to realize.....!!

Friday, January 15

We didn't get to talk to the doctor today, but his nurse called this afternoon to say that they had received our messages and the doctor should be calling us either over the weekend or on Monday. We received some paperwork today regarding the testing next Friday, and it looks like they are planning on doing several tests. The main question we have for him is if the tumor board is recommending surgery at some point, what is the criteria that we need to meet to reach that point? Is it just for the lungs to clear up, or is it dependent on what these tests reveal? I guess we'll know more on Monday!

Now that we have several doctors in the mix, it's hard to keep the appointments straight. Next week he has bloodwork one day, the lung doctor one day, the oncologists one day, and then the Moffitt testing one day...and I think several of those stack up together on the same day! Boy, being sick is a full time job!!

Monday, January 18

Our Moffitt doctor called on Saturday morning and gave us more information on the tumor board meeting. He is a real no-nonsense guy, so I think it's probably better for me to highlight what he said by point:

1. The board felt like Keith would probably be a candidate for surgery in the future, but they need for him to be on Coumidin for at least 3 months for the blood clot, they want his lungs to clear up, and they want more information about the tumor.
2. They said the stuff in his lungs in inflammation from the Bleomyicin, not cancer or infection.
3. They want more testing to see just how involved the Vena Cava is with the tumor, thus the tests next Friday.
4. He said they could not get the current PET scan to load for the board, although it would load for him to view in the clinic. So the tumor board was unable to view the PET. He said he might order another PET scan for next Friday as well. (Hmmm…we'll see how THAT goes with the insurance!)
5. He wants the biopsy slides from the orchiectomy. The board believes that Keith's tumor is pure Seminoma, but they need those slides to confirm that. Apparently that makes a difference in how they approach the surgery.
6. In conclusion, he said he wasn't going to commit to anything until he got the results of these tests. I assume that after the tests he will schedule an appointment with us to go over them. He keeps referring to the surgery as a "big" surgery. When a surgeon says that, you have to assume that what he means is that it is a "risky" surgery. That's what makes us nervous.

So, if he has the surgery, it wouldn't be until at least March. I really want us to all pray that the tumor continues to shrink. If it could shrink down to smaller than 3 cm, they would be less likely to operate (it's at 5 cm now). Also, I think they will do another PET scan before they do the surgery, and if it is small enough, they might be able to tell conclusively if there is or is not any cancer remaining.

Tuesday, January 19

Today has been a normal day. I got up, took the dog out, went in and worked till noon, ate a sandwich, then worked some more. I had to go to the dentist this afternoon, and on my way back I called Keith. He said, "I'm so behind...I've had this meeting and that meeting, and I have the men's thing tonight." He wasn't complaining, just venting a little about being so busy. But...he sounded strong and back where he needs and wants to be.

I remember one day when he was going through treatment looking at him laying on the couch so pale and sick and thinking..."Will we ever have another normal day?" Well, we had one today, and I paused and thanked God for it.

Wednesday, January 20

My enjoyment of normalcy was shattered today, when, at 3:00 this morning our phone rang, and we found out that one of our closest friends in Birmingham had collapsed with a massive heart attack. After struggling all day, he passed away this afternoon. John and Kathy Jones have been friends of ours since we first moved to Birmingham in 1993. We have had many, many great times together, and they were the type of friends that would walk through fire for us, and we would have for them.

They spent a week with us at the first of January, and how we treasure that time now. John's health had been failing in recent years, but we did not expect this. He was only 48 years old.

So, tomorrow we will head to Birmingham to be with our friends and mourn the death of this one that we loved so dearly.

Please pray for us as we travel. Keith will be flying back on Saturday, and I will drive back on Sunday. All the Moffitt tests have been moved to next Friday.

Hug your loved ones close. It is amazing how quickly things can change.

Tuesday, January 26

We are in Dallas today, celebrating Josh's 24th birthday. It has been quite a whirlwind week (remember, a week ago today was my "normal" day....sheesh!). We flew in to Dallas yesterday, and will fly home tomorrow. It has been a great day, though, and I am so glad we made the effort to be with both of our kids on their birthdays. We spent the entire day with Josh, and then took him out for a very expensive steak!

I wanted to remind you that Keith is having the MRI and PET scans at Moffitt on Friday. My prayer is that the tumor will have continued to shrink to the point that they can tell conclusively about the cancer or lack thereof in the tumor. Of course, if it has shrunk to the point that it is below the 3 cm mark, that would be great, too. If we are going through this surgery, I want to be sure that everyone is in agreement that it is absolutely the best course of action!

We see our doctor on Thursday, travel to Moffitt on Friday, and then go back to Moffitt next Friday to meet with the surgeon. Big decisions this week and next...thank you for your prayers!

Tuesday, January 27

We went to see the oncologist today, and he is very pleased with Keith's progress. His lungs seem to be better, and his bloodwork is steadily improving. He was impressed with all the scans that Keith has lined up for tomorrow. He said that Moffitt can get insurance companies to do more just because of who they are, and if they can't get it covered, they will write it off. I still can't believe that he is having another PET scan tomorrow and we haven't had any issues from the insurance. He still thinks that Keith shouldn't have the surgery, but we all agreed that the surgeon will have a much better picture after tomorrow.

The scans tomorrow will be all day! He starts with MRIs in the morning, and ends with the PET scan at 4 pm. We won't know anything regarding the results until our appointment with the surgeon next Friday. Hopefully then he can give us more answers.

So, please pray that the tumor has really shrunk down, but especially that they can have a decision that all doctors will agree on as far as surgery or none. I got this Facebook message from my friend Cathy Eidson Brown, "Be encouraged! Praying for a cancer-free tumor that looks like a raisin! Or, ideally, GONE! Praying & singing 'Great is Thy Faithfulness' as you visit Moffitt on Friday." I love that...a tumor that looks like a raisin! Let's ask God for that!!

Monday, February 1

Keith had all the tests at Moffitt on Friday. It was unbelievable...he arrived at 8:30 am, and finished at 6:00 pm! AND he couldn't eat anything during that time!! He was a hungry boy after everything was over! He said that even though many of the tests were the same ones that he has had before, the level of intensity was greater. It was like they knew what they were looking for and were determined to get the information that the doctor needed. During one of the tests, he was in the MRI tube for 45 min.!! I get short of breath even writing that! It would take LOTS of drugs for me to be able to do that!

He did have another PET scan. Nobody mentioned who was paying for it, so I assume it was either our insurance or Moffitt. I don't think we'll get the bill based on what the Moffitt lady told us, but , if we do, we'll deal with it.

We will get the results of the tests on Friday, at our meeting with the Moffitt doctor. Please continue to pray that the results are clear: either we know for certain that surgery is needed, or we know for certain that it is not recommended. We have a doctor friend at church that has been following Keith's journey, and he is really leaning toward the surgery. His reasoning is that once the surgery is completed, the thing is out and gone...never to rear its ugly head again. I agree, but does that logic offset the riskiness of the surgery? We just need some clear answers.

Wednesday, February 3

Keith talked with the Moffitt folks today to be sure that we got a copy of all the tests for our files and that our oncologist got copies. He was told that the PET scan report was ready, but the MRI scans were still being read. Not sure what that means. It may just mean that the MRI scan reader (otherwise known as a radiologist, I think) was out that day! Anyway, please pray as these tests are being evaluated.

Our appointment on Friday is at 12:30. I promise to update this as soon as we know anything and get home. We are anticipating that the surgery will be on the horizon...just not sure when.

Friday, February 5

I am so sorry that I have not updated this sooner. I literally went from the Moffitt appointment to lighting training at the church, and have just now arrived back home. So, here's the scoop:

We had prayed for a definite answer, and, while it is not the answer we wanted, it seems pretty black and white. The Moffitt PET scan indicated "activity" remaining in the tumor, which the surgeon feel like is cancer cells. So, he definitely recommended surgery. He spent a long time with us, going over all the risks and benefits. It is a very big, scary surgery, that could take anywhere from 5-9 hours. Keith will be in the hospital for up to 10 days, and then will be out of commission for 6 weeks. He said, "This is a very complex surgery. As a surgeon, it's cases like this that wake me up at night thinking about it." You really love hearing THAT.

SO, for now the surgery is scheduled for March 18. I can't lie to you...I am absolutely scared to death over this. We have an appointment with our oncologist on Tuesday, so I know he will weigh in on it. And, of course, everyone has an opinion...do the surgery, get it over with and gone.....get another opinion....wait and do more testing. So, we really need your prayers. I think we have pretty much decided to move forward with the surgery, but I just want to throw up when I think about it. So, pray for peace, and the affirmation from our oncologist that we need to move forward with this.

What a day!

Tuesday, February 9

Well, we met with our oncologist today, to seek his opinion about the surgery. I had a really prayed that if Keith was supposed to have the surgery that our doctor would have changed his mind about it. Remember he was originally against the surgery. We had already decided that if he was still against it that we were going to ask for another opinion. Well, today he came in and the first thing he said was, "So, after looking over the report, I am assuming we are talking about surgery, right?" We spent the next 30 minutes or so talking about the ins and outs and the risks of the surgery vs. the risks of waiting, and at the end of the appointment, Keith said, "I think I need to have the surgery."

I asked the doctor, "So, at the end of 2 very bad months (6-8 week recovery) this whole cancer nightmare will be over and done, right?" He said, "Exactly." He said that he chance for recurrence after the surgery would be minimal.

At the end of the appointment, I told the doctor about my fleece and asked him why he had changed. He said that it had to do with the SUV numbers on the new PET scan. He said that those numbers were too high to ignore. Whatever the reason, we left with absolute confidence that the next step for Keith would be the surgery.

So, March 18 is the day the surgery is scheduled. Please begin praying now for all that surrounds this surgery. It is very intricate, so please pray that God guides the hands of the surgeon. The surgery is Retroperitoneal Lymph Node Dissection. Thanks so much for your prayers. I will update occasionally between now and the surgery, but promise to go back to my daily updates after the surgery.

Wednesday, March 10

Keith's surgery is a week from tomorrow, so I thought I would go ahead and fire this blog thing up again, to get everyone caught up on all that is going on . To be honest, since I last wrote in here, about a month ago, not much has happened. Keith had to go to Moffitt for a couple of tests, including a brain MRI to be sure the cancer had not spread, but everything came back clear.

He is at Moffitt now meeting with the anesthesiologists and having some bloodwork done. He wrote out a list of several questions that he was going to drop by Dr. Sexton's office. Nothing major, just some odds and ends that he wanted to know.

the biggest news is that we just returned from a 10 night cruise. It was wonderful! We had booked it in February of last year, obviously with no idea of all we were facing, and it was such a great time away and time of renewal. We went to St. Martin, St. Thomas, St. Kitts, St. Lucia, and Barbados. So fun!

All in all we are feeling good about the surgery. We definitely know it will be a rough few weeks, but thankfully Keith is so much stronger, so hopefully his recovery will be swift and complete! Plus, I have all you guys praying to that end!

As we approach the surgery, here are a couple of prayer requests:

1. Please pray that when the surgeon gets in there that the surgery will not be as complex as they think it could be. Pray that the tumor pulls away from those critical veins and arteries...and yes, his aorta...so that the surgeon doesn't have to cut it away and have to graft those veins.
2. Please pray for t he surgeon's hands as they maneuver through the nerves in Keith's abdomen. He will be using nerve sparing techniques...just pray that they all work!
3. Pray for Keith's recovery. they have to remove so many things (bowels, intestines, etc) in order to get to the tumor

location. Please pray that all of those things will decide to work again when they poke them back in!
4. Pray that they can get all of the tumor.

I'll update everyday between now and surgery day, and will figure out a way to keep you all updated here during the surgery. It could take 5-9 hours for the surgery. thank you for your support and prayers.

Thursday, March 11

Keith was at Moffitt for over 4 hours yesterday! And in true Keith Martin form, he left his phone at the church, which meant I couldn't reach him! Finally about 3 hours into the appointment he called to let me know everything was okay and that they were just running behind. He had all the bloodwork done and met with the anesthesiologists...they promised to use the small tube to protect his vocal cords!

Everything is on go for next week. He will have to be there at 5 am (I offered to call a taxi, but he wasn't happy with that idea!). The surgery is scheduled to begin at 7:15 am. He is the first case of the day, which I guess is good....the surgeon is not tired, but he might be sleepy!

A friend today asked me what my greatest fear is going into this surgery, and I think it would have to be that because they have to maneuver around so many nerves, arteries and important things, that something would be damaged that he will have to deal with or suffer with the rest of his life. The doctor told us that the greatest risk in this surgery is not the actual surgery itself, but the recovery afterwards...getting everything working again and avoiding infection.

They have scheduled 6 hours for the surgery, so by this time next week it should be over. I'm really ready to be on the other side of this!

Monday, March 15

The surgery is this week. It is hard to believe how fast this month has passed! Keith has had to go to the hospital every day (local hospital, not Moffitt) to get a shot since he has had to come off of the blood thinner in preparation for the surgery. Today he had all the liquid taken out of the lap band in prep for the surgery. He is really hoping he will be able to keep it, as the lap band surgeon told him that if it had to come out they would not be able to put it back in due to scar tissue.

I had several people ask me aver the week end if Keith was okay about the surgery, so Saturday night I ask him, "So, I had 4 different people ask me how you were doing and how you were feeling about the surgery. So, how ARE you doing and how ARE you feeling about the surgery?" He said that while he is not looking forward to it at all, he has a real peace that it is what needs to happen. I guess that pretty well describes me, too. I occasionally have a wave of nausea when I think about it, but I am really ready to be on the other side of it.
So, the countdown begins...!!!

Tuesday, March 16

Today was a really busy work day, as Keith is busily preparing to be gone for an extended time. He has to do fun "prep stuff" for the surgery tomorrow which will keep him housebound, so he will be attending a couple of meetings via Skype! Hopefully he won't take the laptop into the bathroom!! Nothing but clear liquids for him tomorrow...and he had the liquid taken out of the lap band, so he's gonna be a hungry boy!

I was busy as well, but still feel like I have this little cloud over me. About 1 pm I felt like I couldn't move forward. I propped my feet up for a few minutes and just rested and prayed, and in a few minutes I was a bit renewed. I know it is stress over the surgery. So ready to have it done! Keith has had some trouble sleeping the past few nights as well. He will get to sleep okay, then wake up in the middle of the night and start thinking about it and have problems getting back to sleep. Please pray for a restful night tonight for us, and a restful partial night tomorrow night! We have to be at Moffitt at 5 am!!

Wednesday, March 17

This a day full of preparation and anxiety! I know all the scriptures and the songs, and I trust completely that Keith is in God's hands, but I'm still anxious!! The big bottle of gross stuff that Keith had to drink this morning seems to have worked, so at least his bowels are ready, even if the rest of him is not quite so sure. Of course, he is starving, since he is on the clear liquids today, but he'll make it!

Yesterday we received the report from the MRI that he had in February. It was not available when we met with the doctor, so when Keith was there before the cruise he had requested it for our files. It noted a couple of things, but one interesting fact is that the tumor seems to have pulled away from the aorta some more. It is a little smaller (1/2 cm), but it is potentially really good news if they do not have to deal with the aorta.

It's interesting that tomorrow will be the first time anyone has come face to face with this tumor. We have been so dependent on imaging, but tomorrow Dr. Sexton will get to see the little monster. Just hope it's already dead before he gets to it! I get a picture of a video game..."Dr. Wade vs. the Tumor Monster." He has to weave in and out of nerve groups and lymph nodes with his magic sword in order to get to the evil tumor! Maybe I need sleep.

I have a group of college friends that have committed to pray for the surgery at 7:15 in the morning, in whatever time zone they are in. They are from all across the country, including Hawaii, and one is even in Singapore! I have been amazed at the notes and promises of prayer support from all over the country. You will never know how much that means.

I will update here as I know anything tomorrow. I love you all.

Thursday, March 18

7:30 am - Well, I have been kicked out of the prep room while they are finishing the preparations for the surgery. They are going to give him an epidural to aid in pain management both in surgery and afterward. I am sitting here with my buddy Greg Crane and we are watching a beautiful sunrise that Greg has proclaimed as God smiling on Keith today. Keith was in good spirits and so am I. Once he gets into surgery it should take about 6 hours. Will write more as I know it.

10:15 am - The nurse just called from the operating room to say that everything is going well. She said it is going to be a long day, which I take to mean that the surgery may take longer than they had thought. She did say that Dr. Sexton had begun to work on the tumor. Bethany is here with me, and I am so glad. Should have another update in a couple of hours.

2:00 pm - Still don't know any more. They have not called out here since the last time. I am hoping that they are nearing completion, but I have no idea. I asked, but they told me they could not call back into the OR, so all we can do is wait and worry! I'll let you know when we hear something!

2:45 pm - They just called and said that they are progressing slowly. She said Dr. Sexton is making progress on the tumor, but it is very tedious, and will probably be several more hours. Please pray for the surgeon's stamina in this long surgery!

4:10 pm - The nurse just called and said they are about to close him up. I don't know any more than that right now, except that she said the doctor is checking everything out and is about to close. I started to remind them not to leave any sponges in him, but decided that probably wasn't appropriate. We will meet with the surgeon shortly, and I will provide the update as soon as I know more. I can't believe I have been at this hospital 11 hours! It has gone pretty quickly thanks to visits from some sweet friends. Been reading Max Lucado's book, "Fearless," that Keith's cousins sent him. It was a good read today...filled with scriptures about trusting God. More later...

5:15 pm - Bethany and I just met with a very tired Dr. Sexton. His first comment was that the procedure proved to be as challenging as they thought it might be. In fact, when they first opened him up he really questioned whether or not they would be able to get it all out. However, they were able to get it out, and as far as he can tell without any major issues. He said the mass was a quite a bit larger than they had thought or could see from the scans and some of it was in some difficult places, but they were able to get it. He said that there is a small amount of residual tumor left, but for the most part they were able to get it all out. They did a freeze biopsy of some of the tumor and found that it did indeed have some cancer cells remaining. The good news of that is that it absolutely confirms that the surgery was necessary. The bad news is that because of the residual tumor he will have to have some more treatment. That will not be until much later, though, until he has time to fully recover. Please continue to pray for him as the next few days are critical as far as determining his bowel function, fighting infection, and confirming that the surgery went as well as they think it did. He is going into ICU from recovery, and will be there through tomorrow at least. I am exhausted, so I probably won't write any more tonight, but will update tomorrow after I see him.

Friday, March 19

This morning when I got here they had Keith sitting up in a chair! He looks good, just very weak. He gave them a scare last night when his BP dropped to 62/42. They have that somewhat stabilized now, but it is still low, so that needs to be the prayer request for the day. They have a tube going into his stomach to keep it drained, because his bowels are still paralyzed from the surgery. Hopefully in the next couple of days they will be able to remove that and see if those babies will wake up and start working again. We will see the surgeon later this afternoon, so if there is more to tell, I will update later. For those of you Facebook users, Bethany posted a photo of Keith on my page...check it out!

10 pm - The surgeon came by late this afternoon (looking rested and refreshed!). He didn't really give us any new info, just pretty much recounted with Keith what he had told us yesterday. At the end of the visit, he looked at Keith and said, "This is curable, and we are close to being there. There are microscopic parts of the tumor left, and after a final treatment, you will be done." He said we just need to stay with it. After he left, Keith looked at me with weary eyes and said, "There's always one more step, isn't there?" To which I responded, "Yes, and we are going to keep taking them until we reach the end of this nightmare!!" The doctor said they would have the pathology report by the end of next week to know exactly what was left in the tumor.

His blood pressure was a little better this evening. I hope he can sleep better tonight. More tomorrow...

Saturday, March 20

Last night was not a great night for Keith. About 11 pm they found that the epidural that they had given him for pain was leaking. The nurse had to take it out, but wasn't authorized to administer any additional pain meds. SO...from about 11 pm until 2 am, Keith was without pain medicine. From what I understand it was not a happy scene. He's pretty drugged up now. Not sure he's going to remember a whole lot about these days!

So, today's prayer request is for pain management. He is taking the maximum that he can take right now. The doctor said that to give him any more would cause him to start seeing things. While I'm sure we would enjoy talking about that down the road....it's probably not the be thing for Keith to see purple snakes on the wall! He is sleeping a lot, which is good, since he slept so little last night.

They have him up in the chair right now, and are working with him on breathing to keep his lungs cleared. Pneumonia is always a concern after surgery, and it is apparently even more of a concern after this type of surgery. The pulminary doctor said that because of the trauma to the abdomen, the swelling pushes the lungs up, which makes them more vulnerable. So much to think about.

Anyway, looks like he will be in ICU at least until tomorrow. I'll update at the end of the day if there is anything to tell.

Sunday, March 21

Today has been a good day! They came in this morning and took out all of the tubes, cords, and the catheter! Keith has been feasting on apple juice, grape juice and Gatorade! He had not had anything except ice chips since midnight

Wednesday night, so that apple juice tasted pretty good! They walked him around the nurses stand, and while he is moving slowly, he IS moving. His bowels are waking up (that's another one of those phrases I never thought I would write), which is a very good thing.

The talk is that they are going to move him to a room today. We are, however, on hospital time, so who knows when that will happen. He's still pretty drugged up with the pain meds. Drifts off to sleep in the middle of conversations, and sometimes asks some funny things. I'll make notes to "share" with him later!

So, today's prayer request is that everything will continue to wake up and ease back to normal. We have to get all the body functions working before they will let us leave.

6:00 pm - We are in a room! It's a little bitty room, but that's okay. Just feel like we are making progress. He is in room 434. Now that we are out of ICU we can use our cell phones. That's nice, too, as Keith was finally able to talk to Josh.

Monday, March 22

We are moving along pretty well...they took out the pain pump this morning and started on pain meds by mouth. He seems to be handling them well and is not quite so goofy. Everyone seems to be very pleased with the progress. We just need all the "gut stuff" to wake up. That needs to be the prayer request of the day....that all of that inside stuff will wake up and start working.

Poor Keith...first he has testicular cancer, then I have to ask all of our prayer warriors to pray that he can poop! I guess when you go through something like this you definitely have to just throw pride out the window! I just want him back and healthy...so ready to have this behind us!

So...you know how to pray!!!

Tuesday, March 23

Today has been a rough one. Keith is in a lot of pain. The pain is not from the surgery as much as from the gas trapped in his stomach. His stomach is very bloated, and they took him down a while ago for an xray to be sure he doesn't have a blockage. Not sure what will happen if there is. He is walking a lot...I crack the whip about every 2 hours to get him up and moving, as they said that would help him the most.

We made forward progress yesterday, but I feel like we have been standing still or maybe moving backward a bit today. Hopefully tomorrow will bring some relief to him. I have loved the messages of those of you that thought of him in the middle of the night and prayed for him. He was definitely suffering!

Before I go, I do have a funny story for you. Yesterday afternoon I went to use the bathroom in Keith's room. When I went to get the toilet paper, the whole roll came flying off and the little holder went flying across the room. I grumbled a little, but finished up. Little did I know that when the TP flew off, it apparently hit the emergency switch in the bathroom. While I was washing my hands, there were people banging on the door asking me if I was okay. I opened the door to see one nurse at the door and 3 more running down the hall! The one at the door looked a little frustrated with me as she fixed the emergency switch. I definitely had a Steve Erchle moment: "Did I do that...?!"

Thank you for your prayers. Please continue to pray that the digestive system will straighten out. Everyone is very pleased with the progress from the surgery and the incision. If we could get this straightened out, they would probably let us go home.

Wednesday, March 24

3 pm - Good news - the xray showed that there is no blockage, and last night things began to "move!" Keith has felt a lot better today. He's still really weak, but not in the pain that he was yesterday. I am hoping when the doctor sees him that he may decide to let us go home tomorrow or Friday.

He had several visitors today, including some good friends from Indiana. It was great to see them. The visits have worn him out, though, and he is snoozing peacefully. That's nice, as yesterday he could not get comfortable.

So, we are rolling along...still need things to continue to progress, but I feel like we are finally moving forward. I'll be anxious to hear what the doctor has to say this afternoon. I am really hoping we can get home soon. I know he will rest better in his own bed, I'm just not sure that Winnie the dog will understand that she can't jump in his lap!

7:30 pm - Well, shoot! The surgeon came by this afternoon and is still worried about Keith's abdomen being so distended. He thinks it may be lymphatic fluid gathering in his abdomen. He has ordered a CT scan for tomorrow. If there is little or no fluid then we will be fine. If there is a significant amount, then they may have to drain it off. Then if it comes back they may have to put a drain in for a few weeks. This happens when they remove lymph nodes and the seals don't hold properly.

I am so tired...could we please pray for no lymphatic fluid? I would love it if this was a problem that we didn't have to deal with! Needless to say, looks like he's not coming home tomorrow. Hopefully Friday...or at least by Easter!!!

Thursday, March 25

Today has been crazy! I'm so sorry that I haven't written before now, but I couldn't seem to find a minute after we met with the doctor. They took Keith down for the CT scan about 3 pm, but he didn't get back until 4:15! The doctor came by at around 5:30 and said that he did not have any excessive fluid buildup. He has a little bit around his liver, but nothing that he was too concerned about. All in all, he said he is pleased with Keith's progress. He wants him to try and eat a little more, but he thinks Keith will be discharged by Saturday.

When he was talking to us he said, "I really expected to find a lot more fluid than we did. I was very surprised that it was such a small amount." I just grinned and thought, "Hey, you don't know our team of prayer warriors!"

The next big hurdle will be when they get the pathology report back. Not sure when that will be, but that's when he and our oncologist will make the decision about the next treatment. I still have a sliver of hope that the report will come back showing no cancer, but since they did the freeze biopsy at surgery time, that's unlikely. But hey...we can ask...right?!

Thank you all for your prayers and well wishes for both of us. I'm doing okay, just really tired. I'm going to hit the be early tonight to try and catch up a little!

Friday, March 26

Today has been a great day! Keith has really made "the turn" today. He took a shower this morning, and is walking without help.
He has been giving me lots of grief today, so I know he's feeling better! We are pretty sure that they are going to let him go home tomorrow.

We've got a list of questions to ask the doctor when he comes in today, but the big question won't be answered until they get the pathology report back. That question is, "Wha't next?!" We're REALLY ready for someone to say..."It's all over! You're cured!"

I'll write again if we learn anymore from the doctor today.

Saturday, March 27

We are home! Hooray! Took awhile to get here...hospitals just don't get in a hurry when it comes to check out time. Now we just have to convince our little dog that she can't jump in Keith's lap! That may be the biggest challenge yet.

For all of you that have travelled with us over the past 10 days, I want to thank you. Night before last the surgeon was in talking to us about a time, near the end of the surgery, when he was having to resect the most difficult part of the tumor. It was behind the kidney, under the liver, and wrapped around the vena cava. He had someone holding Keith's right kidney while he worked. He said it was very dangerous and with every cut he had to be prepared for profound blood loss. I know (and I think he does, too) that God's hands were guiding him and helped him know exactly where to cut. We believe this man is a brilliant surgeon, but we also know that he was guided by God. We are so thankful that it is over, and want to thank each of you from the bottom of our hearts for your prayers, emails, FB posts, cards, and well-wishes. Keith still has a journey to travel to get back to full health, and then the decision will have to be made as to any more treatment. So, please keep praying!

We love you all...

Monday, March 29

Today has been a pretty good day. Keith's legs are still very swollen, and I called the doctor's office today to ask about it. Apparently the lymphatic system helps to move fluid around the body, so when you remove lymph nodes from the abdomen, it is difficult for the body to pull fluid from the lower part of the body...thus the swelling. The amazing thing is that over time the body will adjust and find another path for the fluid. It will just take time. I'm beginning to see now why they said it would take so long for him to recover. While outside his body looks like it is about back to normal (except for the large incision on his stomach!), the inside still has a long way to go to recover from the trauma.

In case you are interested...we measured the incision today. It is 11" long, with 35 staples! I told you it was impressive!

Tuesday, March 30

We went to our Bradenton doctor's office today to have Keith's blood checked for them to check his INR. Everything looked good, and they checked his legs and said that it is just part of the healing process. He is still moving VERY slow, and any little thing just wears him out. He is making himself get up and walk around the house often in order to try and force the swelling down.

I will still take this over the chemo, because even though he can't move around and is uncomfortable, he at least doesn't feel so awful like he did when he was on chemo. I hate to think about him having to go through that again. But, if it's what we have to do, we'll do it. Still no word from the pathology report from the surgery. Hopefully we will know something about it next week.

Wednesday, March 31

Keith is really having a lot of pain in his right leg. The Home Healthcare nurse came by today (the hospital set it up) and checked him out. His vitals looked good, but his legs are still giving him a lot of trouble. We go back to Moffitt on Friday to have the staples removed, so hopefully we can get some answers about all this pain. He is taking the pain medicine now to help the pain in his legs....the pain from the incision is not bothering him! I know it has something to do with removing all the lymph nodes, I just want someone to look at it and confirm that he is progressing according to the plan.

Please pray for the pain in his legs, and that the fluid will "find its new path" quickly.

Friday, April 2

Keith is having a great day today. We went to Moffitt this morning and got the staples out. The surgeon is very pleased with his progress, and very thankful that he hasn't had any major complications. The pain in his legs is a little better today, but the doctor feels like it will all get better with time.

We did get the pathology report back today, and it showed that there was cancer in several areas of the tumor. Dr. Sexton is going to present Keith's case to the Moffitt Tumor Board on Monday, and then he will confer with our Oncologist about what they all recommend for future treatment. We meet with the oncologist next Thursday, so hopefully then we will know what the next step is. I'm going to remind that doctor that he said that after the surgery this would all be over!! Just kidding...I am just so thankful that we moved forward with the surgery. There is no doubt that if we hadn't done the surgery, that the cancer would have come back.

Another document we received today is what they called the OP Report, and it was a detailed description, step by step, of the surgery. It was 3 pages, single spaced, and was a little overwhelming! I am so thankful that God led us to such a great hospital and such a great surgeon. When you read that document and realize all that was going on that day, it is absolutely amazing.

So, all in all it was a good day. We even went out to lunch after the Moffitt appointment. One of the things they told him was that he needs to be taking in more nourishment, as a part of his blood that indicates that was low. I volunteered to help him on that, as I am always open to take in more nourishment!! He ate a good lunch, and we are going to work on eating more. They also determined that his red count was a little low, so I'm sure Dr. Berry will address that next week.

Have a blessed Easter, dear friends, and thank you for traveling this road with us!

Monday, April 5

I think every time that I write on here that Keith is having a great day, I somehow jinx him! Starting on Saturday, he began feeling really crummy, and was totally wiped out. Yesterday was just as bad, he just really has NO energy, and he has been running a low grade fever in the evenings. The home health care nurse just left, and she thinks that his blood count has dropped more. She called

Dr. Berry's office, and they said to see how he is feeling tomorrow and if he is not better to come in. It's always something....you know? The nurse told him to eat a big steak tonight for dinner!! I'll bet it's been awhile since anyone in the medical profession told you to do that!

All the other stuff is doing better. This is pretty amazing....when he came home from the hospital on March 27, he weighed 223 lbs., and was very swollen. This morning, 8 days later, he weighed 185! That's 38 lbs.! What I wouldn't give to drop 38 lbs in 8 days!! I really feel like if we could get the blood stuff evened out that he would really get a whole lot better very quickly.

Please be in prayer as you think about us tonight, as Dr. Sexton is taking Keith's case before the Tumor Board at Moffitt. That's where all the great medical minds of Moffitt study Keith's case, the treatment and surgery that he has had, and make recommendations on what needs to happen next.

So...today's prayer requests are tumor board and blood!

Tuesday, April 6

This morning Keith woke up feeling better and stronger than he has since before the surgery. He actually did some church work and met with one of our staff members about a mission trip. But...this afternoon...he started having pain again. This pain is through his abdomen and was really giving him a rough time today.

No word from the Tumor board, but we really didn't expect to hear anything. I think Dr. Sexton will confer with our oncologist, and we will find out on Thursday what the recommendation will be.

So, please pray today for these mystery pains. I think it still has to do with things settling in his abdomen...finding their new "home!"

Wednesday, April 7

Today has been a really good day for Keith. He is feeling better, and has had good energy. The Home Health Care folks sent out a Physical Therapist to do an evaluation on him today, and it was really good. He explained some of the mystery pains, and why Keith is having such a hard time getting comfortable to sleep at night. He also gave him a checklist of things to do each day (mild exercises), and challenged him to be walking. He even took him outside and told him how far he wanted him to walk...so what if it is the same distance that I'VE been trying to get him to walk....maybe because the PT said it he'll do it! (or at least I can be more forceful in my requests!!) Ha!

We go to the doctor tomorrow, and hopefully will find out some more pieces to the puzzle. The appointment is not until 4 pm, but I will be sure to update when we get home. Please be praying about this and that Keith can begin to sleep a little better. He just has such a hard time getting comfortable.

Thursday, April 8

Today was a rough one. Not only did Dr. Berry agree that Keith needed to do the additional chemotherapy, but he wants us to start it on Monday, April 19. He will have one round on the 19th, then take a break until Monday, May 24, in order to allow him to direct the Mother's Day Concert, and for us to take a trip that we have had planned with our kids the week of May 16. Then the final treatment week will be the week of June 14.

This treatment will be very similar to the last one - he will have 5 days of treatment, then two weeks off to recover. Every indication is that he will be just as sick this time around as last time. The additional drugs that they use this time will also affect his blood counts. We were VERY discouraged to hear that he is going to have an additional 3 rounds of treatment. I guess we were thinking that since most of the tumor is already gone that it wouldn't take that much to wipe out the rest.

However, the doctor said that the tumor was attached to so many things, that there is no way to tell where or if any was left behind. He said that Keith really doesn't match any of the case studies, so we are really just feeling our way along. He did not want to wait, though, as he said if there are any cancer cells there, they are not just sitting there, but they are already multiplying, so the longer we wait the more risk there is.

Every indication is that this plan of treatment will wipe this out. Of course, we are getting a little weary of being told this, and then there ends up being more. After he finishes the treatment they will follow him for 5 years with periodic scans to be sure nothing comes back.

The big thing we need to pray about is that Keith has not become resistant to the cisplatin, the main drug. There is no real reason to think that he has, but that would be the only thing that could really mess everything up. The problem is that there is really nothing to measure, since the mass is gone.

Please pray for us, and especially for Keith. This news hit him hard today. He knows all too well what those chemo weeks are like, and does not relish the thought of having to go through it again. The only good news is that I feel like we are finally seeing the light at the end of the tunnel. It's just a little further away than we thought it would be.

Friday, April 9

We have had a good day today. I think we have both sort of resigned ourselves to the news from yesterday and are starting to work through it. Now that Keith has realized that next week will be his last one to be free from sickness for awhile, he's starting to compile a list of things he wants to accomplish. One of those things is going to the beach, so I think we may do that one day next week.

Keith's spirits are a little better today. Mine are, too, for those Woodland choir members that are worried about me! We are just tired...tired of the sickness and the treatments and the fatigue, but trying to learn what we can through the journey!

Monday, April 12

Keith felt really good today, and even worked for half the day at the office! He really enjoyed the time to be there and do some planning. I'm not sure he would be pushing himself this week if he weren't going back into chemo next week. He really wants to get as much done as possible, because unfortunately we know what next week holds!

Not much news today. I guess that's a good thing, as there has been a lot of drama the past three weeks!!

Tuesday, April 13

Another good day today. Keith was a little more tired, as he didn't sleep well last night. We were talking at dinner tonight of how nice it would be if the surgery really had taken care of everything and he didn't have to do the treatment again. You really can't imagine how much we are both dreading it! My sweet mother said today, "Well, maybe it won't be as bad this time because you know what to expect." I said, "Thanks for being positive, Mom, but it's going to be awful. We've just got to get through it!"

Thanks so much for the prayers and the messages and cards that we continue to get. You guys that are still reading this are what we all the "long termers!" You are with us long term, even through all of my babbling...and we love you for it!

Thursday, April 15

Keith went to work for a half day today, and he is planning on making an appearance in choir tonight. He is doing great, he just gets tired really quickly. It's hard to believe that the surgery was 4 weeks ago today. They told him it would take 6 weeks to recover, so he is really ahead of schedule! Glad we didn't know at the time that week #5 would bring more chemo!

Please pray for him this weekend. He plans on leading a portion of the service. It's funny, the song "Blessed Be Your Name" was already scheduled, and is such an appropriate one for him to lead! If you don't know the lyrics, here they are:

Blessed Be Your Name
In the land that is plentiful
Where Your streams of abundance flow
Blessed be Your name

Blessed Be Your name
When I'm found in the desert place
Though I walk through the wilderness
Blessed Be Your name

Every blessing You pour out
I'll turn back to praise

When the darkness closes in, Lord
Still I will say

Blessed be the name of the Lord [2]

We have absolutely been living this!

Friday, April 16

Today has been a low key sort of day, but Keith has been SO tired all day. he had an eye appointment this morning, and when we got home he went back to bed and slept for 2 1/2 hours. Then he fell back asleep this afternoon, and went to bed early tonight. I hope he is just catching up from not sleeping very well this entire week. My fear is that his blood is still out of whack. I know they will check it on Monday before they begin treatment. I just can't imagine him being weaker than he is now!

Please pray this weekend about the chemo and whether he needs to begin it now. I know the doctors want to get in there and kill whatever cells are left, and so do we, but I just want to be sure he is physically up to all that it means!

Monday, April 19

Today began the first round of the "salvage" chemo. It really was like a bad version of deja vu! I really couldn't believe that we were back in that room again. This chemo is 5 days a week for 7 hours! It lasts 2 hours longer than the last one! So, Keith gets to open the place up and is still there when they are all ready to go home!

He's already feeling a little yukky from it, but hopefully that will subside with the nausea medicine that he has. We were chuckling on the way home that the last time on the first day he was still on morphine, so he really doesn't remember how he felt!

His blood count was better today. I fed him red meat all weekend! I tried to get him interested in some liver, but that just wasn't going to happen! His red count was over 10 today, and I've learned that below 9 is sort of the breaking point for Keith. This chemo affects the blood, so I am hoping that the counts will stay okay.

Several of you asked for me to post the video of Keith in worship yesterday. You can see it above. Keith was overwhelmed by the cheers and response of the crowd when he came out. He longs to be back doing what he loves.

Well, Day 1 is history...on to Day 2!!

Tuesday, April 20

Day 2 is over, 3 more to go! Keith took his laptop today, and enjoyed being able to do some work while he was there. He's doing okay, but I can tell he's getting weaker. It would be great if the sickness and fatigue would hold off, but I feel like it is inevitable with the Cisplatin.

He said there were a lot of entertaining people in the chemo room today. One especially colorful older woman was trying to get them to implement a happy hour and put scotch in the chemo bags! She also talked about organizing a Bingo game with the chemo patients! He said watching her definitely helped the time to pass!

Thank you for your prayers, emails and kind words. We are doing okay. I am doing okay. With God's help, we're going to get through this. Bless you all.

Wednesday, April 21

So, I called Keith at chemo today to check on him, and he said, "I've decided I want to go to the beach after chemo today. Could you bring my bathing suit and flip flops?" I was stunned, but of course I agreed. We had a wonderful 2 hours on the beach. He walked and picked up shells, and I still can't believe he did it all after Day 3 of chemo! By the time we got home, though, he was feeling pretty rough, and went straight to bed. It was a good afternoon, though!

Okay, I think I need to clarify some things. Apparently after Keith's appearance this weekend, some rumors have run amuck based on some things that he said, or didn't say when he spoke. I had several people stop me today at church wanting clarification, so let me take a minute and give you the facts as we know them:

1. The cancer that they found in the tumor is not a different kind of cancer. It is still pure Seminoma Testicular cancer. Keith said that it is "new" cancer, which confused some people. If it was new, it was the same old cells that have formed into new mass. But it is still the remnants of the 20 in. monster from last year, and it is gone, because it came out with the tumor.

2. The surgeon was able to resect all of the tumor. If you look at a scan right now, it looks like the tumor is completely gone. However, because they found cancer in 3 places when they took the tumor out, there is a likelihood that there are microscopic pieces of it left that are cancerous.

3. Every indication is that these 3 rounds of chemo will be the final treatment. It should mop up anything that is remaining. After that Keith will have periodic scans to be sure nothing is happening with it. This will happen for 5 years. We have been hesitant this time to use the word cure, or cancer-free, since we have said that 2 times before and there have been more steps to take.

4. So, there is not a new cancer. They did find cancer in the lymph nodes when they took them out, but it was the same tumor, not a new form of cancer. None of this was surprising to the surgeon. He said the mass was just too large for the chemo to have penetrated it completely after the first round.

Hopefully that explains everything a little better. We were very overwhelmed to find out he had to go through 3 more rounds of chemo. We just weren't expecting that. We thought maybe one round would do the trick...but no such luck. We're taking it a step at a time, though, and glad to be on the downside of this week! I anticipate that he will be sick tomorrow, so please continue to pray!

Thursday, April 22

The sickness has arrived! It is almost like clockwork! So far the medicines are controlling it, and they even gave him an extra shot of something at chemo today that has helped him, and knocked him out. At least there is only one more day in this round! As we all know, though, then we have to endure the next few days while this is wreaking havoc on his body. He has lost about 8 lbs. this week, and they are not happy about that, so my job is to try to get him to eat...anything...and especially high calorie foods! Life has such irony, huh?! We would have never thought a doctor would ever order Keith to eat lots of calories!

I wanted to share with you a note that I got today from a sweet friend who lost her husband to cancer 6 years ago. He was a pastor, and was diagnosed as a young man. When he died they had four young children. Now that you know a little of their background, here are her words:

The Journey

When I was on the journey that cancer brought my way, I dug into the book of Job to see how God wanted me to react and to see exactly what Job learned about God and His character during his wilderness period. One of the truths that I learned is similar to yours...Our God is trustworthy, and during the times that it feels like He isn't, I have to CHOOSE to believe that He is!

Let me share with you as someone who did choose to trust, He is so faithful. I love My Lord so much. I am deeply amazed that He loves me so perfectly when I am such a mess. But here I am 6 years down the road and God hasn't failed to meet my needs yet! He has met my needs, and then some!!

Thank you for posting your testimony and song from Sunday. Once you have had to walk the road you are on, you never forget how hard it is, nor how precious it is! It is such a contradiction, the hardest times in my whole life, were the sweetest times with My Lord!

I love you both and am still praying. Hang in there....you've almost made it to the end. You can do it!

Laureen

Friday, April 23

Today was a LONG day for Keith. Not only did he not feel good, but 7 hours is just TOO LONG for chemo! He is very weak, and they have given him something for nausea again that has made him sleep, so he has been asleep for the past couple of hours. He had at least put on a couple of pounds this morning. Something shifted in the universe when Keith Martin brought home "Weight Gain" packets yesterday!

I anticipate a difficult weekend, so please continue to pray for us. If he follows the same path as last time, the next few days will be pretty rough, and then he will slowly get stronger. Have I mentioned that I can't believe we are going through this again? Oh, I have? Well, just making sure you knew!

Monday, April 26

Boy, this past weekend was a rough one. Keith was SO sick! We went to the doctor this morning, and found that he was dehydrated. His blood pressure was 70/60! They kept him there and gave him fluids, which has made him feel a little better, but he is still very sick, and unable to eat. He'll go back tomorrow for more fluids.

If it follows the same course, he should begin feeling a little better on Wednesday or Thursday. I am so glad he's got a good chunk of time before we have to go through this again. I can tell you, this weekend we both questioned whether or not there would be a next time. But, I'm sure we will move forward...that's just the fatigue, sickness and anxiety talking!

Interesting fact...Keith weighed 167 lbs. today at the doctor's office. He has officially hit the 100 lb. mark from his all time high weight of 267!

Tuesday, April 27

Keith felt a little better today, but he is still REALLY weak. He actually ate a little dinner tonight, so I am hoping that will help him with his strength. You really can not imagine how rough this past weekend was. I mean, I seriously questioned whether physically he could go through another 2 rounds of this. At least he doesn't have to start round 2 until May 24.

I can tell a difference in my resolve this time around. Last time I was pumping my fists in the air saying, "We're gonna beat this!" While I still believe that, it's harder to pump my fist in the air. We have been told twice now that the journey was complete, only to find that we still had to do something else. I understand the twists and turns, and don't blame anyone, but it is difficult to hit this round of chemo with the intensity that we hit the first round last time. Anyway, hope that makes sense. We are not in ANY way giving up, and if there are 30 more steps, we will take them. But we REALLY hope that this will take care of it.

I need your prayers for strength for Keith. He is planning to direct our choir and Worship Arts Team on Mother's Day weekend (May 8-9). The choir has been working so hard in his absence, and it means so much to him to be there to direct. He will have rehearsals on Wednesday , May 5th (his birthday), Thursday, May 6, and then performances on Saturday, May 8 at 5 pm and Sunday, May 9 at 9 & 10:45 am. It sounds like a grueling schedule, but unless something goes wrong, he should be able to do it. Would you please pray that he can?

Wednesday, April 28

Today was a much better day. Keith still spent most of the day in bed or on the couch, but he wasn't quite as nauseated, and he was more like himself. He even had me go get him a Wendy's hamburger tonight for dinner, and he ate most of it! Of course, right now he's laying on the couch moaning like he ate 4 plates at a buffet!!

I really feel like if his blood counts will hold that he will just continue to get stronger. I think we have pretty much made the turn from the nausea, now we just have to strengthen his body! Hopefully he can continue to eat.

Thursday, April 29

Today was again a little better. He has waves of nausea and achiness, and he is still VERY weak, but he seems to be strengthening. I'm going to try and get him to eat some red meat tomorrow so we can get a head start on the red blood counts. They gave him a shot for the white counts, so hopefully the counts will be okay on Monday.

He is SO tired of laying around, but he doesn't feel like doing anything else. I have had to work, but tomorrow my schedule is light, so I may just put him in the car and drive him around! That's one of the upsides to living in paradise...everywhere you drive is pretty! Maybe we'll get one of the 1400 calorie Chick Fil A milkshakes to try and get some meat back on him! He's down to 163 lbs. Of course, I don't <u>need</u> the extra 1400 calories, but I'm a supportive wife, so whatever it takes, even if I have to drink the milkshake, I will do! :-)

Friday, April 30

Big news...we went out to lunch today! We ran into some friends who joined us, and it was really great! Keith ate a good lunch, and really enjoyed the visit. 'Course he had to take a nap when we got home! That's okay, though, it was a good day.

We finally got our air conditioning fixed today. For those of you that remember, last time during chemo we had what we came to call "chemo Thursdays." For some reason something bad happened every Thursday during the chemo week. Well, this time was our air conditioning. We got it fixed though, just ahead of our 90 degree weekend. I'm a really happy camper...Keith is freezing to death! (We have GOT to get some fat back on that boy!) Anyway I am providing hats and blankets for him!!!

Plan on trying to feed him a steak tonight to work on the blood counts. We will have everything tested again on Monday.

Monday, May 3

Keith was feeling pretty good today. In fact, he drove himself to the doctor this morning so I could work. BUT (of course, there's always a BUT) when they did his blood counts his red count was 7.5. If it is below 8 he has to have a transfusion, SO he goes in for another blood transplant tomorrow! His platelets were low, too (30,000), but they are not going to give him platelets right now. It's really sort of good that he's getting the transfusion, since he has a rehearsal that he needs to do on Wednesday night and Thursday night to get ready for the performance this weekend. Hopefully this will give him the boost that he needs.

He will go back to the doctor on Thursday to recheck the blood. I am SO glad he is not having to go in for Round 2 on Monday. It is going to be great to have the break!

Tuesday, May 4

Keith went in for the blood transfusion today, and he is doing a little better. He is still pretty weak, but I am thinking it may take a little while for it to really give him a boost. Thank you for all of your prayers. You will never know how much you all mean to us.

Tomorrow is Keith's birthday. It's a little staggering to look back on all that has happened since his last birthday. In fact, this time last year he was getting injections in his back for what they thought were back problems. Little did we all know what was actually lurking in his abdomen! One thing I do know now that I am a little more versed in this cancer stuff: If the tumor really had been lymphoma like they originally thought, he probably would not still be with us. The mass was just too big. As rough as this year has been, I sort of understand now why everyone was pretty giddy at the announcement of testicular cancer. We are blessed. We are thankful. We are better for having traveled this path.

If you would like to send Keith any birthday wishes, you can do so via email. He's trying to check them every few days.

Wednesday, May 5

Keith had a great birthday today! Thank you for all the MANY emails, cards, FB posts and wishes. He enjoyed them all. We went out to lunch today, then he came home and rested up for the rehearsal tonight. For those that know him, and especially those who have sung under his direction, you will appreciate this: The concert this weekend is one of the biggest musical programs we do each year. Because of the surgery and the subsequent chemo, Keith has yet to actually rehearse this music with the choir. He has had several very competent people that have worked with the choir, and his associate has prepared the band. So, to summarize....one of the biggest productions of the year...tomorrow night is dress rehearsal....full choir, band, brass, soloists...and tomorrow night is the first time he is rehearsing it! And you know what? It's going to be great! I think all these people have worked even harder because they knew the circumstances and wanted to present it to Keith as a love gift!

The blood transfusion REALLY helped him today. He goes in for bloodwork tomorrow, and I am hoping that if the counts are going to slip that they will go ahead and be low tomorrow so he can get the help he needs. don't want him to bottom out Saturday and Sunday!

Thursday, May 6

Today was pretty iffy. Keith went in this morning and they did blood work. His counts were okay, white count was a little low, but they weren't too concerned. However, when he got home he was completely wiped out. He slept from 10 am til 1 pm, got up and ate lunch and went back to bed from 2-4 pm. I called the doctor's office to be sure his bloodwork was okay, and the nurse said that this is just part of the body dealing with chemo.

I knew he had the big rehearsal tonight, so I jumped online and gathered our Facebook prayer partners together. Within minutes I had confirmations from all over the country that people were praying for him. It was incredible! AND he was stronger when he woke up from nap #2. He made it through the rehearsal and did a great job with it. The program is going to be fabulous! If you are interested, it will be broadcast live this weekend on Saturday at 5 pm and Sunday at 9 and 10:45 am (ET). You can access it at www.woodlandlive.com.

We go to Moffitt tomorrow for our post surgery appointment with the surgeon. I assume it will be our last appointment with him. I'll let you know if we find out any news!

Friday, May 7

We went to Moffitt today for the post op appointment with our surgeon. He was very pleased with Keith's progress, and the way the incision was healing up. We learn new things about Keith's case every time we are there. It seem that he is quite the celebrity around there, and his case "white male, age 51" has been presented at several conferences. Apparently it is rare for pure seminoma cancer to develop into such a large mass. Of the ones that do, only 10 % are still large enough that they have to be surgically removed after chemotherapy. Then only 10% of those have viable cancer in them after surgery. Add to that the fact that testicular cancer is almost always found in men age 18-35 and you see that he is quite an oddity. So, the rarity of Keith's case has made him somewhat famous around Moffitt, even though they only know him as "white male, age 51!"

We met some friends for lunch today, wan while we were there it was like Keith bottomed out. He became really pale and weak. Not sure what was going on , but I drove us home and he slept a couple of hours, and was fine tonight. Please pray with us about the concert this weekend. He will be leading 3 services. I just pray his strength will hold up. I will report in on Monday.

Monday, May 10

The weekend was wonderful! Keith did a great job, and our Worship Arts team was fabulous! His energy stayed up and he made it through all 3 services. I have uploaded the service above, so you can see it if you missed it, or just want to see it again. It is a very large file, so you may have some buffering.

We went to the doctor this morning and he is pleased with Keith's progress. His counts were still low, but he said that is to be expected. He wants to see him again on Thursday to be sure he doesn't need a transfusion on Friday. He said we might need to fill up his tank before the cruise! He confirmed that this particular chemo is especially brutal, and that the fatigue from it is profound. We can attest to that!

Thank you again for all the prayers for the weekend. It really was a wonderful service.

Wednesday, May 12

Yesterday and today have been really low energy days for Keith. He can make it for about half a day, and then he just runs out of gas. On the original schedule, Keith would have been in the second round of chemo this week, and I absolutely can't imagine that! It makes me worried about the final 2 rounds.

He will be leading worship this weekend, and then we are going on a trip with our kids next week. Bethany comes in on Friday, and Josh on Saturday. It will be so good to all be together! Just please pray that Keith's strength holds out and nothing weird happens while we're on the ship!

Thursday, May 13

Today Keith got to participate in the Ordination Council for two of our young staff members that are about to be ordained. One of them was his associate, Andy Botts. Andy has really become a "Ministry Son" to us, and he has done a fabulous job stepping in for Keith during this season of our lives. Keith absolutely loves the mentoring process, and some of you reading this may be those that he helped to mentor in the ministry. It was such an honor for Keith to participate in this special event.

Again, he was able to go and do this little bit, but when he came home he was exhausted. They did bloodwork on him this morning, and while his counts are still low, they weren't low enough to warrant a transfusion. Just please pray for him as he leads worship this weekend, and as we are gone with our kids next week. He just needs a shot of energy!

Saturday, May 15

We are so excited that both of our kids will be here this week. Bethany has already arrived, and Josh will be flying in tonight. I won't be doing any writing here next week, as we will be floating around the Caribbean! Planning on being totally unplugged!! (Oh, and for all you would be robbers...we have some people staying at the house and babysitting Winnie, the attack Yorkie!)

Keith is doing a little better. It is funny how eating read meat seems to give him a bit of a boost. I am hoping he just keeps getting stronger so he can really enjoy the cruise! Please pray that all goes okay next week. I certainly don't want to have to take him to a Mexican hospital!!

I'll post some pictures when we get back. Then, the day after we return he starts round 2 of the chemo. Lovely vacation followed by a kick in the stomach!

Monday, May 24

Our trip with our kids was absolutely wonderful! We had so much fun, and we laughed and laughed! Keith did great on the trip. He usually tired out in the afternoon, but it was vacation, so an afternoon nap was a good idea for us all! The week flew by, and boy, do we ever know how Cinderella felt at the stroke of midnight....that's how it was this morning as we trudged into the cancer center to begin round 2 of the chemo...like we had turned back into a pumpkin!

Because we saw the doctor today, Keith didn't get started on the chemo until 10. His appt. was at 9:45, so by the time he finished at 5 this afternoon, he had been there for over 8 hours! One day down and 4 more to go. This was one of those days today where I really hit a wall. I guess it was the kids leaving, and Keith going back into chemo. The dog and I just sat here and looked at each other today! It really does seem like this is never going to be over. I know that's not true, but finishing day 6 of 15 days still seems like a long way to go, especially knowing what comes between day 10 and 11! (two weeks of sickness!)

Keith's blood counts were low again today, and the doctor mentioned that he might struggle from anemia from this for the rest of his life. I hope that is not the case, because I know he feels so much better and has so much more energy when his counts are up. Thank you again for all of your prayers and encouragement for us. Please pray that there are no long lasting side effects (anemia or neuropathy) from the chemo.

Tuesday, May 25

Today was a really good day for Keith. Yes, he had to sit in a chemo chair for 7 hours, but after it was over he still felt pretty good. He got aquainted with a young man today who was diagnosed with testicular cancer in March. He also has an abdominal tumor, though not as large as Keith's was. He had a lot of questions for Keith today about the disease and treatment, and I think it helped Keith to be able to share his journey. They are planning on talking more tomorrow. Please pray for this young man. 25 years old and facing this difficult disease.

I'm doing better today, too. I know that this weekend will bring sickness, but I also have done it enough now to know that by next week he will be getting stronger and the sickness will go away on Wednesday. He is trying a new nausea medicine this week. It is a patch that he will put on after the last treatment. It should be good, as we have a pharmacist friend who told us that one patch costs $300! Keith will be using a sample that the doctor gave him.

Thank you again for all your prayers and support. It is absolutely what sustains us. Day 2 is finished...3 more days in this round, then 5 in the next, and we are finished!

Wednesday, May 26

Keith is still holding off the sickness. He said he feels like the air is being let out of him, and he is beginning to be very tired, but so far no nausea. We fully expect it tomorrow, but it is nice to have a little extra time. The good news from today is that the nurses got together and examined all the protocols from the many drugs he is taking, and figured out that they could run them a little faster, so today's therapy was 5.5 hours! That's still long, but it makes a big difference.

Since we got out early today, Keith wanted to make a trip to the beach! So we headed out for a couple of hours to sit and watch the beauty. He even did some shell hunting and found a couple of sand dollars. It was a nice little break.

I have the image of us going into a tunnel tomorrow that we will emerge from next week. Thanks for your prayers during the "sick" time.

Thursday, May 27

As expected, the chemo sick arrived today. He is really sick, but we knew it was coming, and we know it will be gone by next Wednesday. It is still amazing to me that the schedule is so predictable. He is trying the new nausea patch, but so far can not tell a big difference.

The good news is that with the way the nurses are running the chemo, it is only taking about 5.5 hours. And one more day in this round. After that, two weeks off and the FINAL round should begin on June 14.

I am so thankful for all of you out there who are praying for us and sending encouragement. I can't believe we are about to head into our 11th month of all of this.

Friday, May 28

Keith was really sick today. Even though we know it's coming, it is still a difficult journey. Tonight I went back and read the Friday entry from the last week of chemo in April. It pretty much described today. I guess the best thing for me was reading the following days, where he slowly got stronger. So, we are "hunkered down" for a really rough weekend, knowing that slowly but surely he will come out of it next week.

I really think the patch is helping him a good bit, but of course he thinks he's never been sicker! When I reminded him of some things from last time he said, "Just let me think that this is the sickest I've ever been. It makes me feel better." Whatever.

Monday, May 31

The weekend lived up to our expectations. Keith was SO sick. Friday night was really bad, but Saturday and Sunday were rough, too. The good news is that today has been a little better. He is still wiped out, but not quite as nauseated. He has bouts of it, but not all of the time. I really think that patch has helped. He's still taking the other medicines, but he seems better than he was last time around. Hopefully he will just keep getting stronger.

I ran lights for our weekend services this past weekend, and our Student Pastor spoke. He said something that really made me think. He told a story of a fraternity initiation when he was in college, where he was blindfolded and one of the other students asked him, "do you believe your faith will catch you?" before they pushed him backwards. He only fell a few feet, but told of the terror of those first few seconds when he didn't know how far he was going to fall. I have thought about that phrase a lot since Sunday. If you had asked me the question, "Do you believe your faith will catch you?" a year ago, I would have said, "Sure...I believe my faith will catch me, no matter what." But since the events that have unfolded in our life since July 14, I would have to answer the question differently. When asked, "Do you believe your faith will catch you?" I would have to answer, "No, I don't just believe it...now I KNOW it. For you see...I have been caught!!" Those seconds (days, weeks) of terror while we were in the freefall have given away to the comfort and peace that can only come from Christ.

Thank you for your prayers during all of this. Tomorrow we will begin month #11. What a journey!

Tuesday, June 1

Today the sickness came in waves. He would feel okay...just really tired for awhile, then he would get really sick. I still think it hasn't been as bad as last time, though. He ate a pretty good dinner tonight, and was able to keep it down.

I feel like we are trudging uphill in a lot of ways. Today I had to tell myself that 2 weeks from Friday all the treatment will be over, and he just has to recover and get back to normal. So ready for that...ready for "normal" again.

Wednesday, June 2

Keith has been doing a lot better today. He slept most of the morning, but when he got up he had a good bit more strength. I failed to mention that he had bloodwork done yesterday morning. His red count was actually up to 11, but his white count was "alarmingly" low. They gave him a Neulasta shot and told him to stay away from people! I think the red count being up is what is making him feel better now that the nausea has subsided.

I want to take a minute to brag on the people of Woodland, our church. They continually amaze us with their love, cards, and gifts. Again, it has been 11 months since this ordeal began, but their passion for us and prayers for us have continued without ceasing. I know there are many of you out there all over the world that are praying for us and for healing for Keith, but I wanted you to know that this body of believers are the hands and feet of Christ to us. I am so ready to be finished with all of this and be back in service with them! Thank you does not seem sufficient, but I know they don't do it for the thanks...they are true servants!

Thursday, June 3

Today has been a good day. Keith has felt good and had quite a bit of energy. I think it really helps that his red count is up. hopefully it will stay that way. In the last round it bottomed out on Monday and he had to have a transfusion on Tuesday. He is scheduled to go in on Monday to have everything checked, so we'll see!

I cooked dinner for us tonight, and he ate a full plate of meatloaf, mashed potatoes, and field peas! He was stuffed! His associate came and met with him for a little while this afternoon. Keith really enjoyed the time to reconnect. If his counts will just hold, this should be a good weekend. We'll see!

Friday, June 4

Keith has hit a bit of a snag today. This afternoon he started running a fever. He doesn't really feel bad, but started having chills this afternoon, and when we checked him his fever was 101. They told us this might happen, and gave us an antibiotic to give him if the fever continued. I tell you, as you have heard me say throughout this whole journey....it's always somethin'!

Two weeks from today it will be over. Oh, sure. he'll still have to be sick for a week or two, but all the treatment will be done!! So ready for that!

Monday, June 7

Today has been a nice day. Keith has felt pretty good all day. He drove himself to the doctor this morning. The bloodwork had mixed results. His white count has come up some, but his red count has bottomed out, so once again he has to have a blood transfusion tomorrow. The nurse told him that it was good that he began the antibiotic when he started running the fever, that if he hadn't he would have probably ended up in the hospital. Lovely.

He went by the office for a little while and said he really felt like a bird out of a cage! He got to visit with Tim (our pastor) for a little while. He is just so ready to be back! Tonight was a real treat...he was able to participate in the ordination service for three of our young ministers. One of them was his associate, Andy Botts. As I have mentioned before, Andy is really like a "son" in the ministry to us, so it was really special for him to be a part of the service.

Good day. Please pray that the transfusion will "pump him up" to make it through the rest of the week. He is planning to lead worship this weekend and really wants to. A week from today he starts the FINAL round!! We are ready to ring that chemo bell...AGAIN!

Tuesday, June 8

Keith went for the transfusion today. It was a long procedure, but he is glad to have it done. Hopefully it will give him more energy to do all he wants to do this week.

Here's a cool Keith story: To pass the time during the transfusion today Keith took several collections of music to listen to. He listened to several of them, and found a few songs that he liked. Then he came across a new collection by Bradley Knight. The last song of the collection was an arrangement of the Gaither song, "It is Finished." Keith listened to it, and when it got to the second verse and the chorus, he started crying uncontrollably...I mean REALLY uncontrollably! Three nurses stopped to see if he was okay! Then, he would regain his composure...start thinking about it again...and start crying all over again. If you are not familiar with the lyrics to the second verse of this song, they are:

Yet in my heart, the battle was still raging
Not all prisoners of war had come home
There were battlefields of my own making
I didn't know that the war had been won
Oh, but then I heard the king of the ages
Had fought all the battles for me
And that victory was mine for the claiming
And now praise his name, I am free.

It is finished, the battle is over
It is finished, there'll be no more war
It is finished, the end of the conflict
It is finished and Jesus is Lord.[3]

He said, "It was like God was saying to me, 'All of those nights when you were so sick, all those hours in the chemotherapy chair, all the battles that you have been going through, I was there, fighting them with you.' Every time I thought about it it just overwhelmed me!"

It is amazing to me the times and places that God chooses to speak to us and reveal Himself to us. Today was Keith's day, and I am so glad it was!

On another note, today I was treated to a special day by several of the women in our choir. For my birthday the choir had given me a "Spa Day," and today was the day! I had a massage, an aromatherapy treatment, a makeover, lunch, and a manicure and pedicure! It was wonderful, and I was so blessed by them! It was a good day!

Wednesday, June 9

Keith has felt GREAT today! It has been so incredible! He went in to work this morning, and worked almost all day. Even when he got home he still had energy to do some things around the house that he wanted to do. I joked with him that if he had to have a transfusion after the next round that I wanted to request blood from the same guy that he got it from yesterday! Seriously, though, the Nurse Practitioner told him on Monday that when your red count is really low, sometimes you don't feel the boost. She said that when your count is not quite so low you tend to see the most benefits. Last time when Keith got the transfusion his count was very low. Yesterday it was just below the point where you have to have a transfusion, and he has really felt the difference!

He may crash tomorrow, but so far today has been great. We just have to get through next week!!!

Thursday, June 10

The past few days have really been amazing. Keith has been almost back to normal! Today he went in for staff meeting, then worked until around 4 pm. He came home for a nap before going back for rehearsal tonight. I am so happy that he has felt so good. It has given us a little glimpse of normalcy before the kick in the stomach on Monday!

Please continue to pray that the blood counts hold. We really want him to be able to do the last round next week. The only good news about next week....a week from tomorrow he'll be ringing that chemo graduation bell again!!

Monday, June 14

Unbelievable! Keith has felt so great over the past few days...then this morning when he went in to start the FINAL round of chemo, they tell him that his platelets are too low and we are going to have to wait a week. We were so bummed! I told Keith, "I bet you never thought you would be disappointed to not get chemo!" The doc said that his platelets are so low, that to give the chemo would reduce them to nothing. So, all of you who are praying for this final round, please turn your prayer support to his blood counts so he can for sure begin this NEXT Monday!

We had a great weekend. Next week is our anniversary, and we thought he would be sick on it, so we made a spur of the minute trip over to Orlando on Friday. It was a lot of fun, even though the crowds and the heat were intense! Now that he is not having chemo, I guess we'll have to do something else special on our real anniversary! Hate that!!

Wednesday, June 16

Keith has had a good couple of days. Once he got over the fact that he "failed chemo," (his words) he decided to utilize this week to its fullest. He worked all day yesterday and had a Navajo mission trip meeting last night, then worked all day today. We had dinner with some friends tonight, so he did come home and take a bit of a nap before this evening. All in all, it has been okay that he didn't go through the chemo, but we REALLY need for him to be able to do it next week, so please pray about that.

If he doesn't get to do the chemo next week, it could affect him being able to go on the Navajo trip, and he really wants to do that. Those sweet people out there have been so faithful to pray for him this year, and the ministry out there is such a passion for him. God knows his heart, and I believe He will make a way for him to go. Please join us in praying about this.

Friday, June 18

The past two days Keith has been really tired. I hope his blood counts are okay. We bought him a big steak to grill tonight, so maybe that will give his red counts a boost! Other than that, he has really enjoyed having the time and energy to get some things done. We were going to go to the beach for a little while today, until we heard that the temp was supposed to be 96 and the water temperature was 90! We decided the air conditioning sounded pretty good!

Please pray for the blood counts, and that he can go ahead and complete the chemo next week.

Monday, June 21

We had a great weekend this past weekend! I know we were bummed that Keith couldn't start chemo last week, but as it turned out, the week and the weekend were really great. I drove up to Gainesville on Saturday for a family reunion. It was wonderful - I saw lots of cousins and aunts and uncles that I haven't seen in a long time. And my mom was there - and I haven't seen her since Christmas! I originally hadn't planned on going, since I thought Keith would be sick.

Then, yesterday was our 29th anniversary (and Father's Day!) We did Father's Day til about 2 pm, then switched to anniversary! We had a wonderful dinner down at the beach. When we came out of the restaurant it was right at sunset. The sunset was beautiful, then we turned around and on the other side of the sky was a beautiful rainbow! We claimed that rainbow as God's promise that this year is going to be great!

Keith's blood passed chemo today, so he is hooked up for the final week! While we know it is going to be a difficult week, I am so glad he was able to go ahead and get started. We just need to get through it and then get him back on his feet! Thank you all for your prayers.

Tuesday, June 22

Keith is really starting to feel the effects of the chemo. He feels really weak and washed out. He's been a little nauseated, but not too bad. He wanted to go to the beach for a little while after chemo today (our doctor's office is just about 10 minutes from the beach), so we headed there about 4 pm. It was still REALLY hot, but we sat under the beach umbrella, and really enjoyed the time for an hour or so. I doubt he will feel like doing that again for a couple of weeks.

I can't believe that the chemo is about to be over. I find it difficult to let myself believe that this journey might be drawing to a close. I want that more than anything, but each time this year we have thought it was over, something else has happened. I guess the thing I have learned the most is just to take things a day at a time, as they come. So, for this week...TWO DAYS DOWN, THREE TO GO...THEN THE CHEMO GRADUATION BELL!! Woo-hoo!

Friday, June 25

Dear ones, I am so sorry that I was unable to update this since Tuesday. The company that hosts this web site had some major issues and had to shut down our access to it. You could still see the site, but I couldn't get to it to make any changes. They have just completed their repairs. I know this week especially that you have been following closely, but I just couldn't access it.

The week has gone pretty much as we expected. He felt pretty good on Wednesday, then started getting really sick on Thursday. Today, He had to be at the Cancer Center at 7:30 am, since they were trying to close early today. they got him hooked up and he was finished by 12:45! The office closed at noon, so it was just us and his 2 nurses to cheer when he rang the chemo graduation bell! that's okay, though, I know all of you were cheering!

He is really, really sick. But it was a great feeling that it is now over! He just has to get stronger from here. Several of you have asked when we will know if it all worked. My joke is that we will know if it worked if he lives to be 80! Seriously, though, they will do a scan in early to mid August to see what, if anything is going on in there. If nothing is happening, then we will wait a few months and do another scan.

Pray for us this weekend. It will be rough, it always is. But Praise God this is the last time!

Monday, June 28

This weekend was really rough. Keith was very sick. He is still very sick today. The nurse this morning told him that the chemo is cumulative, so he is dealing with 3 rounds in his body, and it takes longer to come out of it. He's REALLY ready to make the turn. His red count and platelets were good today, but his white count was really low. They gave him a shot for that, and we don't go back until next Tuesday. This is the first time in this chemo round that he hasn't had to have a transfusion the week after chemo. I'm glad, but I really wish he would start feeling better.

Thank you for your prayers. Please continue to pray for recovery from this round.

Tuesday, June 29

Keith is doing a LITTLE better today. The nausea has subsided, but he is experiencing overwhelming fatigue. He has taken 4 naps today, and went to bed for good at 10. That's okay, though. We can deal with fatigue...he can sleep through that. It was the nausea that was so debilitating. It will be interesting to see how he is tomorrow. If he is not significantly better, I think we will call the doctor to see if we need to come in for a blood check.

It was interesting today. We were talking and he said, "Everyone says, 'at least it is over,' but I can't even think that. I've thought it was over two other times and it wasn't. I don't know when I will really believe that it is over." Of course, I don't think there is anything else they could do to him right now!

Wednesday, June 30

Keith is doing so much better today. He is still very weak, but the nausea is pretty much gone, and he is beginning to make the turn. He even met with some folks this afternoon about the Navajo trip. He is so excited about the mission trip this year. He loves that ministry so much, and they love him! It is looking good that he will be able to make the trip, as long as his blood counts don't go haywire! Please join me in praying about that.

So far so good in the recovery...he's just taking lots of naps, which I've about decided is an okay thing! I've joined him in a couple!!

Friday, July 2

Sorry I missed the update yesterday. Bethany is home, getting ready to leave tomorrow for a month in France. She is doing a study abroad program with Auburn. This week has been a flurry of details trying to get her ready to leave. If you could see her room right now, you would not believe that this time tomorrow she would have all that stuff packed in suitcases headed for Paris!!

Keith is doing pretty well. As most of you know from traveling this journey with us, as we finish chemo there are a series of icky things that he has to go through. It starts with the nausea, and then goes through all sorts of things. Right now he is dealing with the digestive issues, and a low grade fever. Each afternoon his fever jumps up to 100-100.5, just enough to make him feel yukky.

All in all, though, he is making progress. Yesterday he was laying on the bed after he had had a "digestive event." I laid down next to him, and he looked at me and said..."Just so you know, I'm not doing any more of this. If they tell me it's either more chemo or die, I'm ready to go!" Thankfully there is not anything else planned!

Tuesday, July 6

Keith has slowly gotten stronger over the weekend. Saturday he was too weak to go with us to take Bethany to the airport, but by Sunday he was a little better, and he was much stronger by Monday. He went to the doctor today, only to find (surprise surprise) that his red counts are low and his platelets were VERY low (15,000). He went right over to the hospital for platelets, and will go back for a transfusion tomorrow. I am really hoping that this one affects him as well as the last one did. It really gave him a boost! So, 5.5 more hours in a chair tomorrow, but hopefully that will be it!

Bethany made it to Paris, and is really enjoying it so far. We are so thankful for Skype...it's so nice to be able to see her and talk to her every day. She is going to London this weekend to visit with my cousin and see the sights. Yeah, well, it's a rough life!!

Wednesday, July 7

Keith got some new blood today, and can already tell a difference in his energy level...hooray! I was so hoping it would really give him a boost. He had a surprise today - our dear friends Paul and Mariann Strozier surprised him at the hospital. They are from Ohio, but were in Orlando headed to a conference and decided that they couldn't stand being 1.5 hours away without coming to see us. So, they came over for the last of the transfusion, had lunch with us and headed back to Orlando. Such special friends! And I REALLY wish I had a picture of Keith's face when they walked in...his jaw dropped, then he teared up and we all started to cry! Remember last time he was there was when he had the teary experience with "It is Finished"...those people down there probably don't know what to think about us!

Please continue to pray. Keith will be leading worship this weekend, then leaves on the Mission Trip next Thursday. Everything is looking good for him to go, we just need those counts to stay up!

Friday, July 9

The past two days have been really good. Keith went to work for part of the day yesterday. Who would have thought on his last full day of work on March 17 (the day before the surgery) that it would be July 8 before he would be back for good! I told him, "Okay, bubba...vacation's over...this is the first day of the rest of your life!!" Sorry for the cliche', but it really seemed to fit. I pray this journey is behind us!!

Today we went to Lido Key for a beach day. The weather was beautiful, and we had a great time! Keith found a bunch of shells, which most of you know is a great love of his! We both got a little sun, came home, cleaned up and went out for seafood. It was really a great day!

Monday, July 12

Keith went to the doctor this morning for bloodwork. His counts were so-so, but nothing so bad as to need action (ie. transfusion). He has been completely wiped out all day today. He even took two naps! He's feeling a little better this evening. He's not sick, just has overwhelming fatigue. If his counts will bump up even a little bit I know he will feel better.

The doctor okayed him to go on the mission trip on Thursday. He has delegated all the trip stuff out so he can just sit back and enjoy the trip (yeah, I know...those of us who have been on mission trips with him know THAT'S not going to happen!!) Anyway, please continue to pray for him this week as he prepares to go, and I will provide updates as I get them from the trip.

A year ago on Friday, Keith came home from the Navajo trip with what we thought was severe kidney stones, only to find that there was a monstrous tumor in his abdomen. What a year it has been!

Tuesday, July 13

Keith is doing a little better today (or he is just ignoring the fact that he's not). He went to the office today for most of the day, came home and took a brief nap, then went back to the church to supervise the loading of all the supplies for the trip. I'm sure he will sleep well tonight!

Please continue to pray for his recovery for the trip. He is so looking forward to going, and loves those people out there so much (and they love him). Some of our most faithful prayer support this year has been from the community of Black Mesa, deep in the heart of the Navajo reservation. He'll be with them this weekend.

Wednesday, July 14

Today was spent getting things ready for the mission trip. We had to buy Keith some new, smaller pants...he could hardly keep up the last "smaller" ones that we bought! He's very excited about the trip and can't wait to see all of the folks on the reservation. It is truly his passion, and I am so grateful to the Lord that he is able to go this year.

He heads out tomorrow - flying into Albuquerque. The rest of the team will arrive on Friday, and they will head to the reservation (3 hour drive) on Saturday. Then they have to buy sheep (yes, you read that right. Sheep.) for the people in Black Mesa. Our church raised enough money for 15 sheep and two goats. I'm sure there will be lots of interesting stories to come from this one!

Thank you again for your prayers. Keith is getting stronger daily. Just please pray God's protection from any infection. I know it will be a great trip for him.

Saturday, July 17

Keith is having a great time on the mission trip. All the team arrived in Albuquerque yesterday and they traveled to Window Rock this morning. He is very excited about the potential of the week, and just seeing all of the folks out there. I was pleased that when the group decided to go to a park yesterday that he made the decision to stay at the hotel, so he wouldn't risk tiring out before the week began. I really believe he will pace himself.

It is really hard to believe that one year ago today was when Keith was first diagnosed with cancer. He had flown home from the mission trip because he was in so much pain, and they did a CT scan on him a year ago this morning. The doctors freaked out when they saw it, and sent him straight to the hospital. I'll never forget where I was standing on a street corner in Gallup, New Mexico, when our doctor called and told me that my husband had cancer. This year-long journey has been very difficult and yet I can't imagine not traveling this road.

We truly pray that the cancer part of this journey is over, but the lessons learned and the love that we have been shown will last the rest of our lives.

Monday, July 19

The Navajo Mission Trip is going great. They are in the heart of the reservation now in Black Mesa - no phone service (or electricity!) the conditions are pretty rough there, but he loves it! I won't be able to talk with Keith until tomorrow afternoon when they go back to Window Rock. I will report then! Thank you for your prayers!

Tuesday, July 20

I talked to Keith this afternoon, and the trip is going great. They went to Black Mesa on Sunday, and arrived at the little church just as they were beginning their service. When Keith walked in, the people stood and cheered. The pastor cried and hugged Keith and kept saying, "God has answered my prayer." Keith cried on the phone just telling me about it...and of course, so did I. I can't tell you what it means to him to be out there.

Someone asked me the other day if I was worried about him going out there. Of course I am concerned, but the way this trip came together, it is so obvious that God's hand is in it. For me to question that would be to dishonor God. Physically, Keith is doing well. He was really tired on Saturday and Sunday, but has really rebounded yesterday and today. While physically he may be a little weak, I can tell you that his spirit is soaring. This is such a fitting end to this cancer-filled year!

This morning before they left Black Mesa, the pastor and the men of the church gathered around Keith and prayed for him and for the cancer to be gone from his body. He said they prayed in Navajo and English, but mostly Navajo. He said, "I can pretty well tell you that if there were any cancer cells left, they are gone after that prayer service!" Amen and amen.

Thursday, July 22

Yesterday Keith and the group went to the orphanage to give out toys and bikes. The children were so wonderful, and loved all the toys. These children all all Navajo, and they are beautiful. The team visits them every year and takes care bags to the young Minnonite women that work at the orphanage. After the toy presentation, the children were singing songs for the team. It was precious...Keith said there wasn't a dry eye in the house! At the close of the songs, this little girl jumped up and said, "I can't wait any longer...I have to know if it's real!" She jumped up and ran over and started rubbing Keith's head! I guess a white completely bald guy is not something that Navajo children see often!

I am in Texas visiting with Josh for a few days. He's decided this is where he's going to stay, so I'm helping him get all of his car stuff (tags, insurance, etc.) switched over. Bethany is still enjoying Paris. She would really love studying abroad if it didn't have the "studying" part!

Tuesday, July 27

We went to the doctor today, and he seems very pleased with Keith's progress. We will have scans done the middle of August, so please keep us on your prayer list! The doctor told Keith he was one of his only patients to have chemo off and on for a year! It was good to hear him say that he feels like it is over.

I will update this page as I have more news. It probably won't be as regular as it has been, since we have slipped back into our normal lives! I will post when we get the scan dates and of course when we get any results. Thank you so much for your faithful prayers and support for us over the past year!

Tuesday, August 10

For those of you that are still checking on us through this, we received word that Keith's scans will be this Friday and next Monday. The PET scan will be on Friday, and the CT on Monday. Our doctor should have the results back on Friday, August 20, and our appointment with him is scheduled for the following Monday. So, on August 23 we should have some information as to what all is going on inside of him. Please pray with us that all the cancer is gone!

Friday, August 13

Keith went today for the PET scan. We both had to admit last night that we are nervous. We have thought this journey was over several times already, only to find that the cancer was not all the way gone. So, today we are praying for the accuracy of the test, for the accuracy of the radiologist reading the test, and that all the cancer will be gone!!

Friday, August 20

Okay, so I understand some of you are going into withdrawals because I am not updating this each day!! I was talking to my sweet sister-in-law today, and she said, "It's like one of my favorite TV shows has been canceled...I check your blog for updates every morning!" That is so very sweet and very humbling, but I am thankful to say that our life has slipped back into the "normal" range...not a lot to talk about that would be colorful and interesting! But, I will say, after the last year, I know how to be very, very thankful for a normal life.

PET scan and CT scan are complete. We will find out the results at a 9:30 am doctor appt. on Monday morning. We are both a little anxious about it, but pray that our life can stay normal! I promise to update here as soon as we know something!

Monday, August 23

And the PET scan read: "NO CANCER EVIDENT!!" Thank you, Jesus!

When we got to the doctor's office today, we were both very anxious. Dr. Berry came in and said, "So, the scans look good...have you seen the reports?" "No" we replied. "Oh, well, there's nothing there." "Nothing?" we asked. "No, no evidence of cancer, and the pulminary embolism is gone. Everything looks good." I found myself suddenly fast forwarding through the past 13 months with all that has happened to us, and wondering if it could really be possible that it was over. I guess with cancer it's never really "over," but right now this is a really good place to be.

He is still suffering from a few side effects of all of the chemo, so there are still a few things to work on, but those words, "NO CANCER EVIDENT" are a beautiful thing!!

He is officially in remission, and will have another scan in 3 mos, then every 6 mos for 2 years, then once a year. Thank you so much for all of your prayers!

Tuesday, November 16

As I am preparing this book to go to press, there has been a new development. On the routine 3 month CT Scan that Keith had last week, the doctor found a small spot on his lung. He feels pretty certain that the cancer has returned.

At this point, we have a PET scan scheduled at Moffitt, and an appointment with the surgeon that did Keith's surgery in March. Everything has been moving at warp speed since we found out and Moffitt got involved, because they don't want to give this little spot a chance to grow. Right now it is about a half inch, and the doctor thinks it can easily be removed by surgery.

Needless to say, this has knocked our legs out from under us, but there are many things about this that show us God's hand through it. Putting this book together at this time has been good, as we have been reminded again of God's proven dependability. We are not sure what is out there, but it will be an interesting path, and reason enough for The Journey: the Sequel!

What I Have Learned: Lee Ann

As I have been reading over these entries, I tend to be a little overwhelmed at all that has happened over the past year and a half. It's interesting, though, that when you are facing it daily, you wake up and do what you have to do that day, and thank God for lighting the path that needs to be taken that day.

Please know that in no way do I think this journey is over. When cancer enters your life, it is there for the rest of your life. Even in remission, you are known as a "cancer survivor," and the thought of its possible return is always there. However, what I have learned through this portion of the journey is that no matter what we face, God will walk through it with us. Keith could ultimately die of this cancer or another one. He could also get hit by a truck or fall over dead with a heart attack. Or he could live to be 88 like his father did. Only God knows the number of days we will be here.

I am thankful and blessed to have been given more time with this wonderful man that I love. I don't take that for granted at all. We have both come to realize the stuff that is really important and the stuff that is, well, not so much. That is a lesson that can only be learned in the fire. Many of the cancer patients that we traveled this road with are no longer with us. It is a horrific disease that steals life and health, and it is overwhelming how many people are affected by it.

In closing, I want to say thanks for sharing this time in our life. I wanted to put this in book form for my children and grandchildren to have as a written record of God's proven dependability. They will face their own difficulties and tragedies, but I want them to always know that God is trustworthy.

What I Have Learned: Keith

If you've made it to this page of the book, you are much further along than I am at this point. At this writing, I have not read any of the blog contributions. Along with you, I look forward to reading each page, looking back and experiencing the faithfulness of God which He gave us one day at a time.

Am I a different man today – yes. How – I can't really verbalize it all, but here are some insights I've realized. First, the fact of mortality is very sobering. I was in complete shock when I first heard the findings of a tumor and thought to myself – no family history, I wasn't a smoker or alcoholic, didn't live next to a chemical plant. So what did I do wrong? I've pondered this question over and over again. The answer…… nothing. If that question had another conclusion, it means that cancer is a punishment for bad people who've done bad things. We all know that is not the truth. Cancer hits anyone. All of us have cancer cells in our body. They are just dormant. What is it that causes them to "awaken" and spread – that's one that may have to wait till heaven to get answered.

Second, my walk with the Lord must be real and ongoing. The saying is true: crisis doesn't build character, it reveals character. If you wait till you're in the middle of a crisis and try to negotiate a deal with God; that just does not work. Even for me (and I've got a Rev. in front of my name), my faith, beliefs and walk was stretched to the very limits. When you're blood count is screwed up: hemoglobin count below 7, white count below 1, and platelets below 15K (I set a record in that area with my doctor… a new LOW record), you don't have the human strength or desire to grow or pursue anything. Today I am so committed to a daily time with the Lord and long to see growth in others. You see, I know their "shock of life" may be just around the corner and I want desperately to do my part to help them be prepared now.

Third, I am totally convinced that the only thing that matters in life is the time you invest in other people. Possessions, titles, fame, recognition… it's all so temporary. Literally here today – gone tomorrow. When I lead worship now, I look into the eyes of the people in front of me. Not to see if they are singing loud or clapping on beats 2 & 4, but sensing where they are in life that day. Are they coming out of a struggle, facing a crisis today and losing the battle, or needing the tools to face the uncertainties of tomorrow. Everyone in that audience is in some kind of pain, and they've come to church seeking hope. Not music, style, or a verbal slam, but words and an example letting them know – they are going to make it! Today I spend my time and efforts in the office and home encouraging, investing, listening, and impacting the lives God has put in my life. When I die, I want my values and impact to be lived out through my family and friends around me. I want them to be stronger and more purposeful than I ever was.

As a pastor, I've counseled and prayed with many a cancer patient and family member, but never really knew the specifics of what they were going through. I knew the words to say, but I did not identify fully with the situation they were facing and how it consumes every part of you. Today, I am much wiser (and humble too). Here are some of the things I have walked away from this journey with. I want you to read and embrace these truths from a cancer survivor.

1 - The day a person hears they have cancer; that is *the worst day of their life!* Don't just say "I'll pray for you", try to feel their pain as they deal with denial, anger, and the sadness that many people with cancer...die.

2 – The second worst day for most cancer patients is the day a biopsy is taken. For me, it was horrible. I was not "put under", just deadened as I lay on my stomach and the procedure was performed. Think about it: feeling the sensation of the apparatus going into my back, finding the tumor, and literally yanking out a

piece – four times. Just hearing the whispers and groans of the medical personnel-that was the day attitude turned from denial to reality …… I have cancer.

3 – The third worse day for me was the day my hair fell out. I was in the shower and felt something strange on my face… and it was my hair falling out. I turned off the water, dried off, and yelled out to LeeAnn to go buy a set of clippers – NOW. I wanted it off! Afterwards, I looked in the mirror at the newly bald head coupled with the "cancer" skin tone now covering my body and got very depressed.

4 - Know that a cancer patient's time during treatments is horrible. The nausea and tiredness was uncontrollable. For me, I only ate soups for almost 4 months straight - that's all I could keep down. Remember, the cards, emails, voice mails are what keep us going - even when we can't even lift our head off the bed. The notes didn't need to be long or spiritually deep - it just helped to know they cared.

5 - Know that even after a cancer patient hears the words "chemo is done", "remission", or "cancer free", the fact is always in the back of our minds that cancer could return at any moment and we could die. That's not a lack of faith; it's just the reality of cancer. A cancer patient has a keen sense of mortality and quickly re-arranges priorities and schedules.

6 - Most cancer patients feel less of a person when all is done - the treatments just take a huge toll, and sometimes permanent toll, on the body. The self esteem issue is at the forefront of their mind. If you have cancer survivors in your ministry, I suspect they will be some of your best volunteers - use them!

7 - Cancer patients are very open and sensitive to spiritual matters - share Christ with them. They need a real sense that God *allowed this to happen*, not that He *caused it!* All cancer patients are open to prayer at any moment. Pray with them - it re-

connects them to God when they don't have the strength (or desire) to voice it themselves. For me, the countless hours in bed or on the couch gave me the opportunity to deepen my faith and ignite my passion. Derric Johnson sent me a card that summed it up: *Keith, you've always known what you believe; now it's time to see if you believe what you know!*

8 –When offering to assist your friend or family member, it is important to know what to say. Be specific! Don't just say "if there is anything I can do, just call". We won't – we can't even process what's happening today. The entire process it so overwhelming. Offer or tell them something specific you ARE going to do unless they tell you no. For us, it was these offers that meant so much: *I'm going to take care of all your pool chemicals and cleaning for the rest of the year*, or *I'm going to mow your yard every Friday – don't worry about it*, or *I'm going to arrange meals for you Monday – Friday for the next two weeks*. These specific tasks were awesome and we didn't have to organize anything. If you are physically limited, gift cards to restaurants were wonderful for ordering take out. I had one dear friend who called every day. Yes, every single day for almost 13 months. Another sent me a card every week – I knew it was coming. Find something and DO IT.

9 – Even though the cancer patient is the one experiencing the illness, cancer affects everyone in the family. One problem may be getting them to realize it and dealing with what they are feeling. Example: now the family medical history is changed. Cancer is now a permanent part of the list. Did my experience affect my wife and children – greatly! Each member of the family needs that one person who they can open up to… or the friend who will not stop till they do open up and face their own fears and questions. You may be that one or can make that one friend aware of their responsibility. It has to be someone who already has that family member's trust and one who knows that person's make up and personality. There are no blanket

responses – each person is unique in their response and path to dealing with this new reality.

10 – You can't make it through cancer as a patient without two earthly things: good insurance and a great care giver. Yes, we had wonderful insurance and still the out of pocket expenses were in the multiple thousands of dollars. Remember that a care giver's job is just that, a job. Plus it is on top of their ongoing job and responsibilities. LeeAnn had to balance her job, home chores, and now add the time demands for countless appointments for doctors and tests, transportation to these every week, dealing with a spouse with no strength or functionality, do my chores and family responsibilities, assist both children in their ongoing challenges, and try to find time to deal with her own feelings. Oh yes, and find time to rest and refresh her own spirit and heart. I do not know how she did it, but LeeAnn was incredible! She quickly experienced the "for better or worse" part of our vows. But that's what we said – vows! Marriage for us isn't a contract but a covenant. It's not optional when circumstances don't fit your agenda, it's for a lifetime! Bottom line – she stuck with me and I'll never forget it. She is the best!

Summary:
I'll stop here, but leave you with one closing thought: Breast Cancer Awareness Month is October. This was during the throws of chemo for me, and one day, LeeAnn noticed the theme bumper sticker for Breast Cancer - it's *Save the Ta Ta's*. LeeAnn and I decided that we needed a bumper sticker theme for Testicular Cancer, so I am proud to announce and unveil our theme..... *Save the Boys*!

Part 2:

The Journey Home

Wednesday, November 24, 2010

Moffitt worked the impossible and got Keith in for a brain MRI and a PET scan today. they are a little concerned about the brain, as the lungs and the brain are the two places that this cancer travels. We are still praying, praying that the small spot in the lung is the only spot. He also has an appointment scheduled with a thoracic surgeon at Moffitt on the 8th.

Tuesday, November 30

Here is the email that Keith just sent out with the update:

Two weeks ago I had my 3 month follow up CAT Scan at Moffitt. On the 15th we met with our Oncologist and he shared with us that they had found a spot/tumor on my lower left lung. This along with a set of blood work results led him to believe that my cancer was back. This past Wednesday, I had a full body PET Scan and Brain MRI at Moffitt and that diagnosis was confirmed. The bad news is that it has returned and my blood counts indicate the cancer cells are rising; but the good news is that (1) it is Testicular Cancer, not Lung Cancer, (2) it has not spread to my brain, and (3) it is an isolated spot and no other "hot spots" showing up anywhere else in my body.

What does this mean? That is where it gets interesting. Both my Oncologist and Surgeon are totally baffled. Both say there is no way one single cancer cell should be in my body at all. As you know, my case is very rare (falling into only 1% of all cases), and with the new developments, there are yet any case studies to give support and direction to the course of action. First, of course, we need to get the tumor/lesion out. That surgery will be done as soon as possible, BUT after the Christmas production. Then there is probably the normal chemo follow up, but I've already had the "lifetime" dose of two of the drugs normally prescribed. That's the lack of direction for now.

We meet with our Oncologist tomorrow (Wednesday), are being scheduled with the Testicular Cancer Specialist at Moffitt ASAP, and a consult with the Thoracic Surgeon next Wednesday. That's all we know at this point. So keep praying for direction, answers, and a cure for this very cruel disease. Our spirits are good and our faith is strong. The hard part was not sharing this with you, our prayer warriors, before now. We just didn't know what we were facing. Now we know what, we just don't fully know how.

In closing, let me say again that God did not cause my cancer – that is a question still unanswered, but He did allow it. This will be a new chapter in my testing and testimony of faith. He will receive the glory and those who need to see a fellow believer facing trails with faith – will see just that. I am not bitter; mad – yes, fearful – at times, but I want people to see the walk, not just hear the talk. LeeAnn, the kids, and I are still processing all of it, but we are not alone – God Is With Us!

I will let you know what we find out from the doctor's appointment.

Wednesday, December 1

What a day! My range of emotions today has been extreme! We went to the oncologist today, fully expecting that he would say that the next step was surgery. Well, the answer wasn't that clear. He talked to us about how Keith has moved out of the realm of the easy decisions, and that it would take a group of experts to really decide what to do next. He asked that since it was taking so long to get in to see some of the Moffit doctors, would we be open to going to another hospital. "Of course," we said. We had often said that if this ever came back that we would try and go to Indiana University Hospital, (which is the top testicular cancer center in the country) but we weren't really sure how to make that happen, and we assumed there would be a long wait to see someone from there.

Come to find out, that was where Dr. Berry was suggesting. He said, "I would like to get you in with Dr. Larry Einhorn, but he has retired. He is the one who pioneered the treatment for testicular cancer in the 70's, and actually developed the chemotherapy that you have already had." He said he would have the nurse contact IU and see who we could see and how long it would take to get in.

After the appointment we were so discouraged. It is so much easier when the treatment path is clear. It is so tough when no one is really sure which direction to go. Keith and I went to lunch, and probably didn't say 5 words between us.

When we got home, the phone rang, and it was our doctor's nurse. She was very excited that she was able to get Keith an appointment at IU next Tuesday! She asked if there was any way we could make that appointment, and I said, "We will figure out a way!" Then I asked, "What is the doctor's name?" "Dr. Einhorn!" she replied. "I thought he was retired," I said. "So did we, but it turns out that he isn't," she said.

I have to tell you...this man is the top testicular cancer expert in the world. He was Lance Armstrong's doctor. He has been published in major medical journals, and has written books on the treatment of testicular cancer. I really can't believe that we have an appointment with him, much less an appointment in less than a week!

And on top of all of those miracles, we were able to get flights (yes, we are inside of 7 days) for $82 each way! Less than $200 each total! Thank you, Air Tran!

Needless to say, we are wiped out with the range of emotions today, but the IU events were a real confirmation to us both that God is still at work through all of this. Our verse for this segment of the journey is Jeremiah 29:11-13 - *"For I know the plans I have for you," declares the LORD, "plans to prosper you and not to harm you, plans to give you hope and a future. Then you will call on me and come and pray to me, and I will listen to you. You will seek me and find me when you seek me with all your heart."*

Monday, December 6

We are off to Indiana today! Keith says that he may not make it to the appointment because he will probably die when he steps into the 11 degree temperature! That's the low...the high is a balmy 19!! We obviously still feel really good about this choice. I promise I will let you know about the appointment as soon as I can get to a computer to update. At the very latest, I'll do it when we get to the airport tomorrow afternoon. Please pray for us today and tomorrow!

Wednesday, December 8

I am so sorry that I am just now getting to update you on the trip. The appointment ended up taking over 3 hours, which meant we had to sprint to the airport to make the flight, then we didn't get home until midnight...and we were exhausted!! I felt mild guilt at not updating last night, but I knew you would understand. Plus I knew I could write more coherently this morning!

First of all, the experience at IU hospital was great! Everything ran like clockwork. First we met with one of Dr. Einhorn's residents, who took down more information about Keith and his history. I asked a question one time during his part, and he said, "This is a very complicated case. I would rather Dr. Einhorn answer that question." THEN, we met Dr. Einhorn. WOW. He has a little bit of an absent minded professor look about him, but not when he speaks. He examined Keith, then said, "I want to take you down to another room where we can talk about your case." That sounded a little ominous to me, so the walk to the conference room was a long and nauseating one to me! He took us into a conference room that had a table with about 6 chairs around it. He sat across from us, and the cool thing is that when he talked, he leaned across the table and kept complete eye contact with Keith. I wish I had a video of that conversation. As Keith said later, "He is definitely the Einstein of testicular cancer."

So, to make the update a little clearer, I'm going to break it down into the areas that we talked about. He said we had 2 distinct but very different options for treatment moving forward.

1. Surgery - He knew that Keith had an appointment with the Moffitt surgeon today. He said that surgery alone had about a 25% chance of curing the cancer. There was a 75% chance that it would come back, and if it did, we would need to go to option 2, which is more chemotherapy. He said it was definitely and option to try the surgery first, but if the surgery was going to involve removal of a lung or a large portion of the lung, it should be taken off the table. He said that really the only reason to do the surgery would be to avoid the chemotherapy and the side effects.

2. Chemotherapy - which leads me to the second option...high dose chemotherapy. This is chemotherapy in a much higher dose than Keith has had before. He will have to have stem cells harvested from his blood prior to the treatment, as it will kill both the bad and good cells. These will be frozen and "transplanted" back into his system after the chemotherapy. This is a very brutal treatment that will make the sickness that he went through last time look like a walk in the park. But there were 2 very significant things that the doctor said that convinced us that this

is the way to go. First, he said that the high dose chemotherapy triples the rate of cure over any treatment that he has already had. I was blown away that someone was still talking cure. My fear was that we were into the concept of management rather than cure. The second thing is that when I asked him about the mortality rate from the chemotherapy, he said that it is less than 2 %. The highest risk is the risk of infection, but they will monitor him closely through the procedure.

He said that the chemotherapy would take care of the spot in the lung, so if we went that route, no surgery would be necessary. The downside of the chemotherapy (besides going to death's door and back) is the potential for lingering side effects. The drugs can cause neuropathy in the feet and hands, and can cause some hearing loss. He said in most cases these are temporary, but they could be permanent.

So, we have made the decision to move forward with this in Indiana. He will be our doctor, which still blows our mind that we have the very best doctor in the world for this disease. The process started yesterday. We met with a transplant coordinator (called transplant because of the transplant of the stem cells) and walked through the schedule. Dr. Einhorn is very concerned about the rising hcg hormone, so he said we need to start this as soon as possible. They wanted him to stay yesterday, but Keith was determined to come back to direct the Christmas program this weekend! Bottom line...we are going to be spending Christmas in Indiana!!

I have given you a lot of info this morning...to sum it up, he will begin this process on December 20, will come home for 10 days January 7, then will go back January 18 for the second of 2 rounds. He will be completely finished with the treatment by February 7. That in itself is good news, as we thought we might be getting involved in something that would take 6 months or longer.

If any of you have known anyone that has gone through high dose chemotherapy, you are probably weeping right now for what Keith is facing. But I can tell you that I have never felt God's peace any stronger than I did at and after that meeting yesterday. To remind you again, the scripture that God gave me on November 16 when I was crying out to Him was Jeremiah 29:11-13 - *"For I know the plans I have for you," declares the LORD, "plans to prosper you and not to harm you, plans to give you hope and a future. Then you will call on me and come and pray to me, and I will listen to you. You will seek me and find me when you seek me with all your heart."*

Another scripture that a friend gave us that has really ministered to us is Isaiah 43:1-2 - *" But now, this is what the LORD says— he who created you, Jacob, he who formed you, Israel: 'Do not fear, for I have redeemed you; I have summoned you by name; you are mine. When you pass through the waters, I will be with you; and when you pass through the rivers, they will not sweep over you. When you walk through the fire, you will not be burned; the flames will not set you ablaze.'"*

We are about to walk through the fire, but have the promise that the flames will not consume us!

Please begin praying now about the details of all of this, and especially about the long-term side effects, that God will wrap his hands around him and will protect him. We love you all.

Friday, December 10

The past few days have been filled with preparations to spend the next 2 months in Indianapolis. Keith has been busy this week getting all the necessary tests done. Everything from a chest xray to a 24 hour urine collection….which he had to do the day of our Christmas program dress rehearsal! He had to tell all the staff, "That is not Tropicana lemonade in that jug in the fridge!"

Here's the schedule that we will be on: This Friday I will load up the car with everything that we are going to need for a month, including a small Christmas tree and presents, and drive to my mom's in Cleveland, Tennessee. Keith will fly to Indy on Sunday afternoon. I will finish the drive from Cleveland to Indy on Monday. Then the fun begins….

Keith will do prep work on Monday, then will do the stem cell harvest on Tuesday and Wednesday. This is a machine similar to a dialysis machine that will pull his blood out, pull the stem cells off, and put the blood back in. He will begin the chemo on Thursday, and will be in chemo on Christmas Eve and Christmas Day for around 4 hours each day. He will "rest" for 2 days, then they will "transplant" his stem cells back into him. After that, there is a 10-12 day period where he will be sicker than he has ever been, and he will have to check in with the hospital every day. At the hint of any infection, they will admit him to the hospital. At the end of that period we will come home for 10 days, then will go back mid January to do it all again. We should be home for good around the second week of February.

It is amazing how one by one, things have fallen into place. We have a place to stay. Our kids are coming up there for Christmas. We have people to babysit our dog and our house. We have seen so many amazing things…some of them big and some very small, but all have reminded us of God's dependability. Here are some cool stories:

Moffitt Doctor – This is a big one: After the PET scan, our doctors wanted us to see a medical oncologist (Dr. Fishman) from Moffitt. Dr. Sexton's office made the request and told us we should hear from them on Monday or Tuesday, November 29 or 30. We didn't. When we met with our Bradenton oncologist on December 1, he said, "We can't continue to wait on Moffitt. Are you open to going somewhere else?" You know the rest of the story (or if you don't read below). Of course, at the time our doctor had NO idea that we would be able to get in with Dr. Einhorn. That was the miracle that happened later that day. ANYWAY…when we got back on Tuesday night at midnight, we had a computer generated reminder call for Keith's appointment at Moffitt the next day. I called that next morning to find out what the appointment was, as we didn't have it on our calendar. Sure enough, they had scheduled an appointment for him with Dr. Fishman, but for some reason we had not been contacted about it. I thanked them, but canceled the appointment.

Here's the significance….if that appointment had been on the table at the Dec. 1 appointment with our oncologist, we would not have pursued the Indiana route. We would have waited until the Moffitt appointment to see what doctor Fishman had to say. God just kept anyone from contacting us so we would move forward with the call to Indy. Wow.

Mom's ticket – My mother was schedule to fly here for Christmas. I bought her ticket with Allegiant air back in the summer, and "accidentally" bought trip insurance on it. I was frustrated about it at the time, but after I did it there was no way to take it off. Thankful for it now…I changed her flight to a spring visit!

Keith's ticket – Keith is flying to Indy on Sunday…that's Christmas week! For some reason, we were able to get him a nonstop flight from Sarasota into Indy on Sunday afternoon at just the time we needed it for $82! Unbelievable!

Dr. Berry – When Keith was in this week for his tests, our Bradenton oncologist, Dr. Berry told him, "You need to realize that Dr. Einhorn is a living legend in medical oncology. You are with the best." We realize that and are so thankful.

So, pray for us as all of these plans come together. There is a massive amount of "stuff" to do this week. We are going to Disney on Sunday and Monday…a trip we have had planned since September. We started to cancel, but decided that it would be nice to get away for a couple of days together before all the fun begins. We love you all, and you will never know this side of heaven how much your prayers mean to us.

Friday, December 17

What a whirlwind week! We had a wonderful couple of days at Disney. The weather was cold, but the decorations and lights were so pretty, and we really do turn into kids again every time we go! Where else can you see a life-sized gingerbread carousel?!!

Tuesday we came back to reality, though, and hit the ground running. My run came to an abrupt halt on Wednesday when I had the mother of all stomach viruses! I was flat on my back for 24 hours almost to the minute! I was better yesterday, and slowly got back onto the Indy treadmill! That little setback means that I am leaving tomorrow instead of today, but that's okay...it meant that I could enjoy the 75 degree weather we are having today before heading to the frozen north!

Keith has begun taking the Neupagen shots to boost his bone marrow before they gather it next week. Please pray for him this weekend. They are giving him 4 times the dose that he has had in the past, and in the past it has given him back pain. They told him that he could expect some rather sever bone pain as that marrow pumps up. He going to be telling his story as part of Tim's message this weekend and there's no telling what he'll say if he's full of morphine! Ha! Seriously, it's an important weekend for him, as he wants to share with our folks all that is going on.

Monday, December 20

We are here, and I have one thing to say....I MISS FLORIDA! When I got about 20 miles south of Indianapolis, it started to snow. Just a little at first, but by the time I got to the hotel it was like a snow monsoon!! We got the truck unloaded in t he snow...we were soaked by the time we finished...and COLD! I asked one of the employees if it was supposed to snow all night and she said, "Oh, it's just supposed to snow an additional 3 inches or so...it shouldn't be too bad." Yeah. Whatever. I miss Florida.

The place we are staying is very nice. Definitely more than a suite hotel...it's more like an apartment. It's very spacious and clean. It's not home, but definitely a place we can call home for a few weeks.

Tonight the Lord sent us 2 special couples. We met them in the lobby as we were coming in tonight. They are both here for transplants, I didn't really understand what was being transplanted, but they have pancreatic cancer, and the transplant has something to do with that. One couple is from Georgia and the other from Alabama, and they are all strong Christians. It was like a taste of home, especially when one of the men looked at Keith and said, " Roll Tide!" They later brought us some cookies from a little party that they had today. We are learning that most all of the people in this hotel are transplant patients. Keith rode with a lady on the shuttle today that is waiting for a liver transplant. She has lived in this hotel for 7 months! The people here have formed their own community, and it is really special to see the relationships. The couples we met tonight are on the transplant list, waiting for organs to be donated. Their names are Don & Deb from Georgia and Larry and Patsy from Alabama. Larry and Don are both waiting for transplants for the same thing. Would you please add these special folks to your prayer list?

Keith had the special port put in today. That was about all of the excitement. They will begin harvesting the stem cells tomorrow. We have hit a small snag with our insurance. Nothing has been denied, but they are refusing to expedite the approval process. I'm going to tackle all of that tomorrow, and would appreciate your prayers.

I had a great visit with my Mom over the weekend, and was able to have lunch on the way today with a sweet college friend, Cathy Brown. She's the one that originally gave us the chemo chicken soup recipe that we have shared with so many people.

In case anyone is interested...it is 1020 miles from our driveway in Bradenton to this hotel....and I'm tired of driving!!

Tuesday, December 21

Today the weather was better...a balmy 34 degrees. The snow is really pretty, and I will say that they had the roads and parking lot cleaned off by mid morning. We had to be at the hospital at 8, and Keith spent the entire day plugged up to a machine that pulled the stem cells out of his blood. We have to go back tomorrow to do that again, and they will probably start the chemo on Thursday.

The kids have arrived, and we are looking forward to a couple of days with them. They are expecting a big snowstorm here on Christmas Eve...so the White Christmas is looking promising! The insurance stuff is in the process of working out. Please keep that on the top of the prayer list. If the insurance doesn't come through, we'll have to put Keith's photo on a pickle jar in convenience stores for donations! Just kidding...I feel confident it will all work out.

Wednesday, December 22

Keith was back on the stem cell collecting machine today. They need to get at least 2 million cells (preferably more like 5 million) in order to proceed with the transplant, and yesterday they were able to get 200,000. Keith said, "Shoot, I didn't even make the T-ball Team!" They gave him a shot last night and tonight that is supposed to aide in the production, and looks like we will be back at it tomorrow. Whenever he reaches the magic number, they will start him on the chemo. Not sure if that will be Friday or Christmas Day.

It is so great having Josh and Bethany here. We all sat in Keith's little cubicle and talked and laughed today. I think tomorrow will involve several card games. In a really weird sort of way, this is a good experience. The four of us being together with nothing to do but be together and hang out with Keith while he has treatment is great. It is a precious time, and one we will always remember.

We had a really neat experience happen today. We set out tonight to find a Walmart. We had a burned out headlight and Keith wanted to get it fixed before he got sick. We also had several things to pick up, so we googled the closest Walmart and then set out to find it. It took longer than we had thought to get there and the traffic was heavy (and it's cold), so we were all (especially Keith) a little frustrated when we got there. We went around to the auto department, and Keith went in to ask about the light. They had it in stock, but could not install it until tomorrow. Keith decided that he and Josh could install it, so he bought the light and came back to the car. Bethany and I went into Walmart and left the master mechanics there in the parking lot trying to figure out how to install the headlight, which turned out to be nearly impossible since they didn't have any tools.

In a few minutes, a man came out that was one of the Walmart mechanics. He offered to help with the headlight, and in the process he and Keith started talking. Keith told him we were from Florida, and he said, "Really, what part?" Keith said, "Bradenton." The guy stopped what he was doing and looked at him and said, "That's where I'm from." Come to find out, he was raised in Bradenton and moved to Indy several years ago. When Keith told him why he was here, the guy told him that he was a kidney cancer survivor, and had been in remission for a couple of years. He said that when they moved up here, his marriage was in trouble, and then he found out he had the cancer. He said he just went to church one night and the pastor prayed for him and he just knew God was going to take card of him.

By this time they had the headlight finished, and Keith asked him if he could pray for him. Immediately the man hugged him and said, "yes." Keith asked him his name, and then prayed for him, and for his marriage and his health. Afterward, the man said, "I really needed to have something good happen today. My attitude has been terrible. Thank you."

The reality is that Keith also needed something good to happen. His heartbeat is ministry, and it really charged his battery to be able to minister to this man. It was definitely a divine appointment.

So, please pray that tomorrow they can get all the stem cells that they need. We are ready to get on with the chemo. Not ready to begin it, but ready to be through it.

Friday, December 24

The first round of chemo today lasted from 8:30 this morning until 4 pm this afternoon. Not all of that was chemo time...some of it was meeting with doctors and having labs done. Tomorrow should be a little bit shorter, but we will probably be there from 8 am - 3 pm or so. Quite an interesting way to spend Christmas. Our kids are being very flexible, though. We are going to open presents tomorrow afternoon, and Christmas dinner will consist of hamburgers cooked on the George Foreman grill!

We watched the Woodland Christmas Eve service tonight, and it meant the world to us when Tim had the congregation clap to say hello to us and that they were praying for us. We truly miss everyone.

One of the doctors that came by today told us more about the procedure and all the side effects. He said that after the first round they will potentially start trying to rebuild the bone marrow during the time we thought we were going to get to come home. So, we may not be coming home for awhile. Sure was hoping for a little sunshine break, but if we need to stay, we will. We just need to get through this.

Another cool story...our nurse from the stem cell collection, Candy, shared with Keith on Wednesday that her daughter has had some severe health issues. That was about all that was said, but that night Keith was having trouble sleeping, so he began to pray for Candy and her daughter. The next day he told Candy that he had prayed for them, and was asking more about her daughter. She teared up when he said that to her, and explained that her daughter had severe allergies and hardly ever left the house for the first 10 years of her life. She shared the story of all that they had been through, and thanked him so much for the prayers. Yesterday when we left she hugged him and you could tell she was so thankful that someone cared about her and her daughter. It was really a cool thing. It is amazing what all people have in their lives. Everyone has a story.

It's 10:30 pm, and still no snow. They say it is coming, but none yet. There's plenty on the ground, so not getting any more is fine with me...it's still a white Christmas! Merry Christmas!!

Monday, December 27

The weekend went well. Keith was in chemo Saturday and Sunday until about 2 pm. Saturday we came back and opened presents with the kids, and then had a Christmas dinner of hamburgers prepared on the George Foreman grill. Keith really felt great through it all, and we were so thankful. The effects of the chemo started to set in yesterday, and have continued through today.

He is really, really fatigued, and a little nauseated. He has slept most all day today and has had no appetite. They say that's okay, though, as long as he keeps drinking!

Dr. Einhorn came by today and talked with us for quite awhile. He said that because they were unable to harvest all the stem cells that we would not be able to go home during the break between chemo. They will have to go right back into boosting the bone marrow, in order to do the second round of chemo within 3 weeks of the first. We were sad that we are not going to be able to go home, but thankful for all the folks that are helping us out in Bradenton.

We received two bits of good news today. First, the hcg hormone that was at 750 when he started is now at 450. That means it has taken a hit just from the first round of chemo. That's good news. They said they normally don't see it drop that much so quickly. The other news is really big....the insurance is covering all of this!! We got confirmation today. That was a huge answer to prayer!

Please pray for Keith as these side effects are setting in. Also, our kids are driving back to Birmingham tomorrow, so please pray for safe travel for them. Bethany is going back to Auburn, and Josh will fly out of Birmingham on Wednesday going back to Dallas. It has been so great to have them here with us.

Tuesday, December 28

Keith had a rough night last night. The nausea from the chemo has started. The thing that is a little different this time from our last chemo experience is the fatigue. He is sleeping up to 18 hours a day. The doctor says that's okay, though. At least when he's sleeping he's not sick!

He has done pretty well this evening, even ate a chicken pot pie (don't worry, it was a frozen one, not homemade like the one I made last chemo that made him so sick!!) We are also managing the nausea pretty well with drugs. They don't mess around here...you would not believe all the medicines he is on. He is on 4 different antibiotics!

The stem cells go back in tomorrow. The process takes about 45 minutes, but he will have to have fluids afterward, which takes about 4 hours. We are at the hospital every morning from 8:30 til around 1 pm for him to get fluids and antibiotics and will continue that schedule for another 2 weeks. They said the infusion of the stem cells should be uneventful. Just please pray that they take hold and start producing, especially since we have to harvest more in a couple of weeks.

We met another couple, Daniel and Shannon, that are gong through the same procedure. Daniel looks to be around 30 years old, and is from Alabama. He is about 2 days ahead of us, as he had the stem cells put back in yesterday. Keith went in and met them on Sunday and prayed with them. They are very sweet and very young to be going through something like this. Please add them to your prayer list.

We saw the sun for the first time since we arrived today! It was still only 19 degrees, but for some reason it doesn't seem as bad when the sun is shining. It was pretty short-lived, though, as the clouds rolled back in this afternoon.

Josh and Bethany made it back to Alabama without any problems today. Josh will fly back to Dallas tomorrow. It was hard to let them go today!

Wednesday, December 29

WOW...what a long day! We arrived at the hospital at 8:15 this morning and finished at 6:00 tonight! They had to do the re-infusion of the stem cells in two batches, one this morning and one this afternoon. They also upped his fluid to 3 liters, so now the fluid takes 6 hours for infusion. So, for at least the next 2 days we will be there for 6 hours. I told them that was fine, but on New Years we had to have him back here by 1 pm to see the Bama game!

He is doing pretty well...the nausea is being controlled by the drugs. He is still really tired, but we are at least underway now that the cells have been put back in. He should be really sick by about Saturday.

Also, I know several folks have asked about visits from Indiana people, or friends that you have up here, so I wanted to give you this information...from this Friday through about next Wednesday, he will have no immune system and can have no visitors. We would love to see you, but please plan any visits around those days. I'm going to guard him like a mother hen! Feel free to email me if you have questions about coming. You can access my email above.

The biggest prayer request right now is that all of this will do what they want it to do. We want his immune system to be destroyed. We want him to stay free of infection. We want the stem cells to take hold and re-energize. And finally we want him to recover to the point that we can reharvest the stem cells for the next round. Love you all, and thank you for your prayers!

Thursday, December 30

Keith has had a really good day today. He slept really well last night, and has had more energy today than in some time. I think it is the calm before the storm, as they say by this weekend he will probably be feeling pretty lousy. That's okay, though, we'll take it! Not a lot of news from today. Just 6 hours of fluids!

It has been a dark, rainy day in Indy today. The temperature is up to around 45, which made all the snow melt. This is the first time I have seen this place without snow, and it's a little drab! The lovely snow mountain behind our hotel is really just a big dirt mound! It was nice, though, not to be freezing when we went to the car this morning, and to not have to scrape ice off the windshield!

Friday, December 31

Okay...HERE WE GO! Keith's counts dropped drastically from yesterday to today. His white count is at .8 and his platelets are at 6000. For those of you medical types...that is not a misprint! The good news is that is what they want to happen. That means that the chemo is doing what it is supposed to do. Needless to say, he got a transfusion of platelets today, and we have started all the neutropenic precautions. He has to wear a mask if he leaves the room, no one but us in the hotel room, all food has to be prepared in here, no fast food or take out (stop laughing, those of you that are familiar with my love of cooking!) He can't drink tap water and can't have ice from the ice maker. He has virtually no immune system right now, and it will get worse, as they expect that he will be at 0 tomorrow. This should last until the middle of next week or so, then he should begin to pull out of it.

He is feeling rough today. His blood pressure dropped really low today (66/40), so they pumped him full of fluid and told him to stop taking his blood pressure meds! By the end of the treatment time it had come up to 116/74. So far the nausea has been managed. We just need to pray that God will place a bubble of protection around him and protect him from any bugs that are out there.

It warmed up to 57 here today, but it is still VERY gray! These folks all think it's spring...still a little chilly to me! We are looking forward to a quiet New Year's Eve...probably won't even make it till midnight! Keith's beloved Alabama plays at 1 pm tomorrow, and the nurses have all promised to have him finished with treatment so he can be back here in time for kick off. He's just fussy that he has to watch it on "fuzzy" TV (no HD) I think he is a little spoiled!

I was poking around on our insurance web site yesterday and found the page that lists all of our expenses for the year. As you may remember, Keith had the major surgery in March, chemo in the summer, and now this little excursion. Year to date, our insurance has been billed over $433,000! Our portion has been around $5000. So thankful for good insurance and good doctors!

2010 has been an interesting year. This time last year we thought we were pretty much finished with the cancer stuff. Who knows what 2011 holds, but I know God will travel with us, and we are so thankful for each of you and your friendship, support, and prayers! Happy New Year!

Saturday, January 1

We are rolling along today. White count is at .5 and platelets dropped to 5000. They gave him a platelet transfusion again today. He has really avoided the terrible side effects to this point, and even the doctor commented today that he was impressed with the way Keith's body was responding to the chemo. The indication is that it is going to get worse before it gets better, but we are pleased that so far he is holding the worst of it off.

He is feeling pretty rough this evening, but we think it may have been to much excitement with the Alabama game! He put on his Mark Ingram #22 jersey, and even managed a few big cheers during Bama's 49-7 win!

Not much news today...fluid infusion and college football has been our day. It's a little weird to not be able to get out and go anywhere. Not been a problem so far, but I think we may get a little stir crazy before he is "released" to the public again (probably in about 10 days.) It's all good, though, as we are really enjoying the peace and quiet. I am also still working, so my days will be plenty busy beginning Monday.

Monday, January 3

Things are getting a little tougher. Keith is really wiped out, yet not nauseated, which is great. His platelet count dipped to below 4000 again today, so he had to have a transfusion. Dr. Einhorn came by today, and he is pleased with Keith's progress. The HCG hormone came down to 108 this week (started at 750, down to 450 last week) and that is really good news. That tells them that the chemo is working.

Our main prayer request now would be for his bone marrow to build up enough for him to be able to harvest the stem cells again before the second round of chemo. His physician team - Dr. Einhorn, Dr. Abinour (Stem Cell transplant doctor), the nurse practitioner assigned to him and the case manager - will all meet tomorrow to discuss which direction to go after he comes through this round. Please pray for them as they make these decisions. Also, continue to pray that Keith will be protected from any long term side effects. He has begun to have neuropathy in his feet that is very irritating.

Tuesday, January 4

This has been a rough day. Keith felt okay when we got to the hospital this morning. When they did his bloodwork, they discovered that his potassium and something else was really low. They had to add these infusions on to the end of his usual ones, and both of them have to run slowly...so we were there from 8:30 this morning until 6 pm! In the meantime, Keith started getting sick. He threw up once at the hospital and has been sick once since we got back. I think he let his stomach get too empty. Food at the hospital is not really great, so maybe he'll do better now that he's back with my home cooking (Progresso soup! Ha!)

Keith just saw that I was updating this and said, "Be sure they know how horrible today was." So...from the horse's mouth...it was bad.

Thank you for all the sweet emails that I have received today. When I am writing this, I can't think about the number of people that are actually reading it or I get a little overwhelmed. Thank you that you allow me to be open and honest about the trials and joys of traveling this road (and yes, there are some joys). Thank you that you endure my fragmented sentences and misspelled words. It's a type of therapy for me, and plus I realize from putting the journal together for the book that down the road it will be a great source of encouragement, seeing God's hand and leadership through it all.

No word on the physician team meeting. I'm not sure that we will hear anything for several days. They will wait to see how Keith recovers before they will make firm plans on what is next. Please pray now that he continues to strengthen. It's about time for the counts to start coming back up. Everyone is different, but they could start back up any day now.

Also please continue to pray that he will be able to harvest enough stem cells for the next round of chemo.

Wednesday, January 5

Okay...today has been one of those days where I feel like I've been nibbled to death by ducks. Keith's infusion was extended again, so we were there for 6 hours. There were several family issues and work issues that I had to take care of, and none of them went the way I had planned. Think I'll go to be early tonight!

Okay, enough about me...Keith is really, really wiped out. I had to take him into the infusion center today in a wheelchair. He doesn't really feel horrible, but has NO energy. His red blood count is starting to be affected now, so he's getting a double whammy. I talked with one of the doctors today about "the plan," and it seems that nothing can be firmly decided until they see when his counts come back up and what they come up to. They should start coming back up by this weekend. Please pray to that end.

It is supposed to snow here tomorrow night, so we will be driving in snow to the hospital on Friday. Yipee. This Florida girl doesn't do so good driving in snow. Maybe we'll just take a "snow day" that day! Somehow I don't think Dr. Einhorn would look to kindly on that!

Thursday, January 6

Another long day today. Keith was at the hospital from 8 am until 5:30 pm. The main culprit for these long days is low potassium and magnesium. Both of these have to be infused over 2 hours, and can't be infused together, so he has to stay up to 4 hours longer than normal. He is starting on an oral prescription for these, so hopefully they will start coming up.

He's still very weak, and is enjoying the wheelchair rides up to the infusion center. Please note, Greg Crane...that I am the one pushing the wheelchair!! (I had some issues pushing Keith in a wheelchair at Disney World so Greg had to take over!) Anyway, aside from the extra infusion it was pretty much business as usual.

We came out of the hospital today to snow. We are supposed to get some more at some time in the next few days...REALLY makes me miss Florida! I'm ready for some Florida sunshine and the Florida beach! A friend of mine from New Albany said that I'm getting payback for all the times I called and ragged him about the 70 degree temp in Florida when it was 20 degrees here! Okay, so maybe I did that once or twice...but this little stint is confirming that I am now a Floridian!!

I had a lovely surprise today from Toni Wampler...a former Woodland member that has moved to Indiana (just south of Indy). She showed up with homemade soup and the best homemade brownies I have ever put in my mouth! I can assure you when got home in the snow this evening that the soup REALLY hit the spot! So thankful for all the many people who serve us in so many practical ways. There are folks watching the house and the dog, more folks that went over and took our Christmas decorations down, and many others waiting in the wings to help do anything that we need! We love you all.

Friday, January 7

Well, they made the decision to admit Keith to the hospital today. Hold on...I hear that collective gasp! It's not quite as bad as it sounds. When someone starts to come out of neutropenia, they will often run fever. Keith started running a fever last night. His fever got up to 101.7. The odd thing is that even with his fever that high, he really didn't feel bad. That is a sign that it is a neutropenic fever. He was still running fever this morning, and the "rules" are that if you start running a fever you have to be admitted. The odds are that the fever is neutropenic, but on the off chance that it is an actual infection, he would get really sick really quick with no immune system. The fever was down all afternoon, but they still wanted to keep him overnight. I anticipate that he will come home on Sunday if he doesn't have any issues. His white count has started coming back up. We just need to pray that it continues.

This has been a rough day. Earlier I mentioned meeting Daniel and Shannon, another stem cell transplant patient. He's a young guy, maybe 30 years old. He's about 2 days ahead of Keith in the process. Anyway, today he had to have a platelet transfusion, and he had a very serious reaction to them. It was really scary and touch and go for awhile, but he came through it. They admitted him, too, for observation overnight. We have spent a good bit of time with them over the past 2 weeks, so it was really tough to see them go through all of that. Please continue to pray for this young couple.

Then...when Keith finally got to his room, he is actually on the Bone Marrow Transplant floor. Tonight I went across the hall to get Keith a cup of ice, and there was a big family out in the hall, and all of them were in tears. I feel certain that they had just lost a loved one. I came back into the room, and all the events of the day were just too much and I busted out crying. (And those of you that have seen it know that it's not pretty when I bust out crying...I don't just tear up!) Poor Keith had no idea what was wrong with me. I finally got it out, along with, "I hate hospitals!" Most of the people on this floor have leukemia or lymphoma and the transplant process is very difficult and they are very seriously ill. I don't really hate hospitals...I'm just ready to be through with all of this.

It snowed all day today. That was sort of nice, in that we opened the blinds on the window in the room and watched it snow. I guess we got about 2", but by the time I came back to the hotel the roads were clear. Please continue to pray for the rising counts. We may actually get a hospital break for a few days next week before they start getting him ready for the stem cell harvesting again.

Monday, January 10

Lots of good news today! first of all, Keith got out of the hospital. His white count is up to 2.5, which is great! that says that the stem cells have taken hold and are reproducing and doing their "stem cell thing." Secondly, he has actually been released from the first round of chemo! You probably don't realize it, but we have been at the hospital for a minimum of 4 hours every day for the past 21 days! He will still have to go in the rest of the week to get the neupagen shots, but that should be a quick run in. I'm so thankful to have a little break...we are both exhausted.

Finally, the REALLY good news. One of the things that created such a sense of urgency for Dr. Einhorn was the rising HCG hormone that Keith had. You may remember that it went from 120 in November to over 300 in early December to 750 when we came and started treatment. They check the hormone every Monday. The first Monday after chemo it was down to 450, the following Monday it was at 115, and today...it was **15**!!! That is really great news, and shows that the cancer has taken a direct hit with the chemo.

Keith is still pretty wiped out, and is having lots of "digestive issues." Please pray for his continued strengthening and that he will be strong enough to harvest the stem cells again.
We are expecting 5 inches of snow tomorrow. We all know how I feel about that. Yuk.

Tuesday, January 11

We were only at the hospital for an hour today! They checked his blood, and his white count is up to 8.5! Hooray! AND they have given us tomorrow off. We don't have to start the neupagen shots until Thursday. Keith is also definitely feeling better.

We got a ton of snow today. It is very pretty, but I'm ready for it to be gone. We have a one day break where we can get out and do something, and we are snowed in!! It's okay, though, just thankful for the break.

The next prayer focus should be on the collecting of the stem cells. That will begin next Monday. They would love for him to be able to collect in 2 days, but we are not sure that will happen.

Several of you have asked about the young couple, Daniel and Shannon. He was fine the next day after the platelet scare. He has been released for his break, and they were going home to Alabama. He will start his second round next Wednesday.

Wednesday, January 12

This has truly been a lazy snow day for us! We slept late, then heard on the news that it was 22 degrees out with 30 mph gusts, which meant blowing snow and a wind chill of near 0, so we decided to stay put in our cozy little suite! We watched a movie this afternoon, then Keith napped and I caught up on some work.

He is feeling pretty good today. He had a good bit of energy this morning that waned a little this afternoon, but he is just tired, not sick, which is good.

We heard on the news tonight that there is snow on the ground in 49 states today. All except Florida! While we wish we were there, we realize that this is definitely an experience that we haven't had in a long time and don't plan to have again...so we are trying to enjoy the snow. but don't get excited...there will be no snow angels!!

Tomorrow starts the neupagen shots - 1 in the morning and 1 at night. They will also do his bloodwork to be sure everything is holding up.

Thursday, January 13

Not a whole lot to report today. We went in for bloodwork and neupagin shots this morning, and they found out his magnesium was low, so he ended up getting to stay for 3 hours! Hopefully that will be it, though, as tomorrow he just has to go in for the shots.

This afternoon our Ohio friends, Paul and Mariann Strozier came over for a visit. It is so great to see them, and we actually went out to dinner for the first time in over 3 weeks! It was great!!

Four more neupagin shots tomorrow...please be praying that they build up those stem cells!!

Monday, January 17

HOORAY! Keith was able to harvest 1.6 million stem cells today! That's enough for the second transplant. That is such a miracle! He doesn't have to go back to harvest more...in fact, the doctors are not sure when to tell him to come back! He is not scheduled to begin the chemo until Friday, since they expected it to take four days for him to harvest. We assume they will bump it up a few days, though. He talked to his coordinator today, who said he would have to talk with the stem cell doctor to plan out what was next, so we should just sit tight tomorrow until we heard from him. No problem!!

I've started calling Keith the 1.6 million dollar man! Te celebrate tonight we went to a wonderful steak house here in downtown Indy. I think it was the best steak I've ever eaten!

Please continue to pray for the next chemo round. We know what is ahead of us, but just knowing it is the final round makes it a lot easier to bear!!

Tuesday, January 18

We ended up with the day off today. Our coordinator called this morning and said that Dr. Einhorn had approved for Keith to start the chemotherapy tomorrow. So, I worked a good part of the day, and Keith took it easy...I mean it's hard work creating 1.6 million stem cells!!

The weather today was "rainy and warm," quoting the local weatherman. The high was 40...that's warm up here!!

The success yesterday really gave us both an emotional boost. We talked a lot today about when we would get to head home and things we wanted to do when we got there. Starting the chemo early means we can finish up and head south a little earlier, we hope!

Please continue to pray about the side effects of the chemo. Keith is already experiencing some neuropathy in his feet. They say that in most cases it is temporary, so please pray that it ends soon and that it is not worsened by this final round.

Wednesday, January 19

Today started chemo again. Keith is still feeling okay, which made it easier. Daniel and Shannon were back, too, and Daniel came over to visit this afternoon and he and Keith compared war stories. I know I have said it before, but this young man is 27 years old. I can't imagine having to go through this at such a young age. But, as my sweet mother always says, "You do what you have to do!"

The BIG news today has to do with the HCG hormone. If you remember, when Keith started the count was over 750. It has steadily moved down, and today it was at 5.9! The goal is to get it to normal, which is 3 or below. 5.9 is sure a lot closer than 700, and it really shows that the chemo is working. We thank the Lord for these little bursts of light and hope.

We are braced for another snowstorm tonight. Depending on which news channel you watch, we could have anywhere from 3" to 10". Most seem to agree that it will be around 6". Boy, I promise if I can just make it back to Florida that I will stop taunting my northern friends during January (the temp in Bradenton was 70 today!!) You guys that live up here can remind me of that next January!

Two more days of chemo and then the fun begins. Please pray that the side effects will be minimal, but most of all that this will wipe out any cancer that is remaining.

Thursday, January 20

Today was relatively uneventful. Keith is starting to feel the effects of the chemo. He is very tired, and is like his battery is running down. His counts have started down, and his red count seems to be affected more this time. It's all part of the process, though, and he will probably have to have a transfusion. I remember the first time he had to have a transfusion, I was really worried...now it's just a part of the journey. I'm just thankful for the folks that have given the blood!

We ended up with about 4"-5" or snow. It was really pretty when it was falling today. Tonight the low is supposed to be 1, with a high tomorrow of 12, with wind chills of up to 10 below. You really can't imagine just how cold that is!

Tomorrow is the last day of chemo. He will go in for fluids over the weekend, then will have the stem cells reinfused on Monday. It is so nice to be moving toward the end of our Indiana adventure!

Friday, January 21

Today was the coldest day in Indianapolis in 2 years! The air temp was -2 and the wind chill was -15! It was SOOOO cold! The nurses at the hospital are always waiting to hear my comments on the latest weather event. Today I told them I finally understood the purpose of a garage (after scraping ice and snow off of our car in -2 degree weather)! In Florida garages are for storage...here they keep your car warm and dry...wish we had one!

Well, the chemo is finally over. It was nice to see that last bag drip out today. Of course, we are far from finished! The stem cells will be reinfused on Monday, then we have to go through the whole netropenic stage again. He is really starting to feel the effects. His counts were okay today, which is good. I am hoping they don't really start to dip until after Monday.

I feel like today marked a milestone...the end of the chemo. Now we just have to get through the next couple of weeks and head home for recovery!

Monday, January 24

Stem cells are back in! The reinfusion went fine...the gave him IV Benadryl and Ativan beforehand, so he was REALLY loopy during the entire event. The reinfusion only took about 30 minutes, but they have to have a roomful of people when it is happening...a doctor, nurses, and the medical techs, just in case something awful happens. It didn't, though, and he was actually feeling pretty good this evening. The weekend was a little rough, though. Yesterday he really felt bad and kept getting dizzy when he stood up. We finally made it to the hospital and they did the positional blood pressure on him. It was low but okay when he was lying down, but when he stood up it was 69/43! They stopped everything and gave him an extra bag of fluids, and he was better after that.

I went to a little get-together on Saturday that the two couples that are waiting on transplants (the ones I mentioned before from Alabama and Georgia) had put together. It was for transplant patients and their caregivers that are staying here at the hotel. Keith couldn't go, but I went down, and there were quite a few people there. These two couples, the Littles and the Russells, have been here for over 4 months now waiting on multivisceral transplants. That means they will get small intestine, liver, stomach and pancreas. Both men have a very rare cancer that requires this procedure. They met here and have become great friends. They are also working to provide support for this community here. When I hear some of these stories I am reminded again how blessed we are that Keith has a cancer that can be cured. Anyway, please add Don Little and Larry Russell to your prayer list. If they get called in for transplant they promised to let me know so I could let all of you know to be praying for them during the surgery.

The temperature today hovered at around 33, and believe it or not, it seemed bearable! Not that it was warm or anything, but there wasn't that bitter cold that takes your breath away when you walk outside. It will be short-lived, though. The cold should be back before the weekend!

Tuesday, January 25

Keith had a really good day today. The only thing that went awry with his counts was his platelet count. They were down to 8000, so he had to get a transfusion. Other than that all he needed were the fluids today. He felt good all day, and looked great. I know we still have the worst of this round ahead of us, but it is nice to have a good, strong day.

It was sunny here today, with temps in the lower 30s. Indianapolis really is a nice city, and I bet it is a fabulous city in the spring! We just managed to spend time here in its worst month! No more snow scheduled for a few days, but hey...we are becoming snow experts!!

Trudging on!!

Wednesday, January 26

Counts are down! White count is at .5, and platelets and red count are holding steady. The white is the significant one, so he is now neutropenic. In case you don't remember, that means no tap water, ice from the ice maker, and food from restaurants. Until the counts come back up I have to prepare food for us here. That's okay, though. I sort of know the ropes this time around.

Today is Josh's 25th birthday. I can't believe my baby boy is 25 years old! He had to work today and had class tonight, so I'm not sure if he got to celebrate! He was born on Super Bowl Sunday in 1986...we watched the Bears and the Patriots while I was in labor! For those of you that remember, that was the Refrigerator Perry "Super Bowl Shuffle" year.

We are at Day +2, which is how they monitor post stem cell transplant. We will have to be at least at Day +11 or 12 before they will release him, and it could be longer than that if his counts go wacky. Please keep praying that he stays on course, and most of all, that the chemo has killed all the cancer.

Thursday, January 27

Today has been more of the same...4 hours of fluids and an additional 2 hours of potassium. His platelets hit a new record low today at <4000, so he had to get a transfusion. He was feeling really rough this morning, but after he got some fluids at the hospital he perked up some. It is amazing how quick things can change and the counts can drop.

Tomorrow is Day 40 here for us. Everyday except 2 we have been at the hospital for at least 4 hours. Today I read the passage of scripture in Matthew 4 that speaks of Jesus' 40 days in the desert. The commentator that I read said that for the people of Israel the desert was a place of testing, encounter and renewal. That definitely describes our time here. It's humorous that my spiritual lesson came from comparing this place to a desert, since up until now we have called it the frozen tundra! It is definitely a place of testing, encounter and renewal, though, and we are thankful for it.

Please continue to pray that he counts will recover and his body will be protected while they are so low.

Friday, January 28

Same song, second verse today...4 hours of fluid and an additional 2 hours of Magnesium. These long infusions make for such a long day! Today Keith slept for about 3 hours when we got back to the hotel. He is so wiped out, and we are both so weary. I feel like we are in that last leg of a marathon (not that I have ever run one, mind you!). The end is in sight, but each step is really difficult.

I am trusting that by this time next week he will be feeling a whole lot better and we will be making plans to come home!!

Monday, January 31

Hooray! Dr. Einhorn came in today and said, "I have great news. For the first time since you arrived here your HCG hormone is normal!" We are thrilled! It shows that the chemo has delivered a knock out blow to the cancer. We won't know anything for sure until after the scans, but it all looks promising!

The really big news here right now is the weather. We are expecting a major winter weather event (and in this part of the country, when they say major, we're talking MAJOR!) On the news just now they said, "the biggest ice storm we have seen in decades is now hitting Indiana." Aren't we lucky to be in the big middle of it? We are expecting 1-2" of ice and up to 10" of snow. We are under a winter storm warning until Wednesday at 7 pm...yep, that's right....48 hours of winter weather!

The good news is that because of the storm, they have admitted Keith to the hospital. His counts are still really low, and they didn't want to run the risk of something happening and us not be able to get him back to the hospital. So, he's all tucked in there, and I am at the hotel. Not really sure when I will be able to get back over there. It is supposed to be really cold after the storm...high of 15 on Thursday! We are just taking it a day at a time.

At least this whole ordeal will give us lots of interesting memories of this blessed 2 months!

Tuesday, February 1

So, here we are in the big middle of one of the worst ice storms in Indiana in decades! It really is unbelievable! I was iced in at the hotel today and couldn't even get to the hotel. I started to try one time, but my car is completely encased in ice. Then I talked with Keith on the phone and he said, "Don't try and come...the last thing we need is to have to deal with an accident up here." So I stayed at the hotel and he is at the hospital.

The last time I spoke with him he was doing pretty well. Just all the usual things that he has to deal with. We really need to pray that the counts start to come back up. Last time they came up on day +11 from the transplant. Tomorrow is day +9 on this one.

Hopefully I will be able to get there tomorrow. We are supposed to get some snow tomorrow, but I we are not going to get as much as they originally thought. I really hope this is our last "winter weather event!"

Wednesday, February 2

I finally made it to the hospital today about noon. No, I didn't drive. Our hotel has a shuttle, so I took it. The roads are pretty bad, but the biggest thing is that I can't imagine getting my car de-iced! I'm going to take the shuttle again tomorrow, so I'll worry about the car on Friday. (When the high temp is 15!)

Keith is doing pretty well today. They have off of everything except the antibiotics and fluids. The doctor told him he would probably get out of the hospital on Friday, and would continue out patient. His counts have not started back up yet, but hopefully they will soon.

The big news is that they have ordered the CT scan for him on Friday. Dr. Einhorn wants to review it before we leave to see just what all the chemo has done to the disease. That makes me nervous, but I'm ready to move forward. I assume that we will find out the results of the scan on Monday. Please pray about that!

Thursday, February 3

Keith's counts still haven't budged. They are encouraged about something called the differential. They said it told them that he has 100 healthy adult white cells. That rattles my mind to think about it. But, apparently they are encouraged by this. They have promised him that he won't have to watch the super bowl in the hospital, but it may be Sunday morning before they release him. Even then, we will still not be "released" to come home.

The CT scan is tomorrow morning at 9 am. I get a little nauseated when I think about it. I just hope that Dr. Einhorn is pleased with whatever he sees on it. We won't have any information on it until Monday. I really expect next week to be the week that lots of things start happening, but who knows? I thought this week would be, too.

The adventure of the day today was when my cousin and her husband came to help me de-ice the car. It was totally unbelievable! I really wish I had taken pictures. The ice on the hood of the car was 2" thick. We finally got it cleared off, then some men in the parking lot helped Greg push it out. There was probably 3-4" of ice around the tires. Greg was raised in Michigan and said that this is the worst he has ever seen. I could have NEVER done that by myself! Still not sure if I will drive tomorrow, but at least I have access to the car if I need it, and that task is complete. Because the one thing I know is that it would be a LONG time before all of this melts! Thank you, Greg and Brenda!

Friday, February 4

So, Keith had the CT scan at 9 am today. At 11 am I was out getting him some ice and saw Dr. Einhorn in the hall. That is unusual, as he usually isn't on the unit except on Mondays. As I was going back to the room, I saw him coming toward Keith's room, and my blood went a little cold. He came into the room, smiled, and said, "I've got good news for you. The CT scan came out completely normal!" We all cheered and jumped up and down (okay, I jumped up and down, Dr. Einhorn didn't.) He said that the scan was so clear that Keith didn't even need a followup PET scan, and that he could do follow up visits at home. He doesn't need to see Keith back here for 6 months! then I said, "So you are saying that it worked?" He smiled and said, "Yes, it did. I told you that the cure rate for this was 90%." Keith said, "Yes but up til now I've fallen into that 10%!" Not this time, woo-hoo! We were thrilled that he came to tell us himself. To get that news from Dr. Einhorn was the best gift we could have received!

His counts are still low, but starting to move a little. His white count is at .5 (was at .3 yesterday). Since he didn't take a big jump, it looks like he will be in the hospital through the weekend. We'll get to watch the super bowl on the little hospital TV. That's okay, though. The news from today certainly made up for that! Then SOMETIME next week we will be headed south! And we are ready!!

I have to tell you, there is no way in the world we could ever thank all of you for your prayers, emails and support. I am completely in awe of the number of people who are praying for Keith around the country and even around the world. We got a letter yesterday from a church in Gulfport, Mississippi. It was a letter from their prayer ministry letting us know that they had prayed for Keith last Wednesday night, and then had the signatures of all the people that prayed for him. I have no idea how they got Keith's name or if we even know anyone at that church, but they took the time to pray for Keith, and that is so incredible. This particular segment of our journey has really taught me a lot about prayer.

This time around, the passages of scripture that I have clung to are Jeremiah 29:11 and Isaiah 43:1-2. The other night I was reading the full 43rd chapter, and the last verse has been what I have carried with me the past few days: *"Yes, and from ancient days I am he. No one can deliver out of my hand. When I act, who can reverse it?"* We are blessed and thankful.

Saturday, February 5

Before I head to the hospital, I thought I would do a Saturday morning edition and update you on some things. Last night, Keith called me to relate a really cool story that happened after I left, and I wanted to share it with you. You remember Daniel and Shannon, the young couple that have been going through this treatment alongside us? Well, Daniel got good news from his CT scan as well. His cancer is a little different from Keith's, and he has to take oral chemo for the next few months, but overall the treatment was very successful for him. And, being a young whipper-snapper, he has bounced back quicker, so his counts came up to the point that he was released yesterday.

Before they left, they stopped by Keith's room to tell him goodbye and it turned out to be a really special visit. We realized a few weeks ago that Daniel and Shannon weren't married, and Keith jokingly kept offering to marry them in the hospital. Last night Daniel asked him if he would consider coming to Birmingham and marrying them. Of course Keith said he would love to. That opened the door for Keith to talk to them very seriously about some spiritual things and beginning their marriage on a firm foundation. He said it was a great conversation.

Back a few weeks ago after Daniel had the bad reaction to the platelets, Keith talked to him pretty bluntly. He said, "Man, you almost died. Is there anything spiritually that you need to get in order?" Daniel assured him that his spiritual life was in order, but it was interesting that last night he told Keith that he felt like Keith had been brought here during this time for him.

Of course, all of this made Keith's day. I have to say, I have been very, very, very proud of him through all of this. Henry Blackaby in *Experiencing God* says, "Find where God is at work and join Him." That is absolutely what Keith has done over the past 50 days. Most people would have curled up and whined (I think this is what I would have done), but Keith has kept his eyes opened every day for the opportunities that were there to share God's love. I think of the auto guy at Wal Mart, the Apharesis Nurse, and all the clinic nurses.

He has also been a great encouragement to the believers at the hospital. When he would find that someone was active in their church, he would question them about their church and what they are involved with. The nurses that come in humming, he asks what they are humming and more times than not finds out that they are on their church's praise team. Then he questions their favorite songs and encourages them to keep serving. All of this with a white count of .4 and red count of 7 (in case that doesn't mean anything to you, it means he would be really fatigued.)

Okay, I've rattled on enough, but I wanted to share this before I headed to the hospital. I talked to him this morning, and his white count is at 1.2! That's great news, and means that we should be able to go soon.

Oh, and by the way, we woke up this morning to 2" of snow and still snowing. Unbelievable. Supposed to get 4" today and more tomorrow. I am very weary of this! I hope when we come back in 6 months for the return appointment with Dr. Einhorn that we will have nice weather and can redeem this city! Every time we have been here the weather has been crazy, even our early visit was with record-breaking low temps!

Saturday, February 5 - 6 pm

Okay, I know I already wrote today, but something neat happened today that I have to share. First of all, Keith is doing really well today, and looks like they will let him out of the hospital tomorrow (so he doesn't have to watch the Super Bowl on the little TV in the room!) He will have to go back on Monday, but if everything goes well he could be released for good on Monday! We will still have to pack up, but if all the pieces fall into place, we hope to be on the road on Wednesday. We will stay a couple of days with my mom in Tennessee, and then hopefully be home by next weekend. We also need the weather to cooperate. We got 5" of snow today and I think there is more on the way!

Anyway, back to the story. Today I went to get a cup of coffee on the BMT Unit. They were out, and since I feel like I own the place, I went over to the clinic to steal some of their coffee. I told one of the nurses what I was doing, and she told me that there was a young man in the clinic treatment room that had been asking about Keith. I went in and met Doug, a sharp young man with testicular cancer that Keith had met several weeks ago. Doug is on the first leg of his journey, going through the BEP chemo right now. He and Keith got aquainted one day and sat and talked while he got chemo and Keith was getting Magnesium. He hasn't been back since them. Keith has asked about him several times, but their schedules never overlapped.

Anyway, to make a long story short, I gave him the update on Keith and somehow we started talking about our churches, which led to talking about Mission Trips, and I started telling him about the Navajo Mission Trip that Keith takes every year. He was very interested and said he is a youth leader at their church, and every year they take a mission trip somewhere. He stopped by Keith's room this afternoon before he left and they swapped information. I really believe he may try and work with Keith to take a group out to Navajo (and Glenn McIntyre, if you are reading this....he is an architect and the other youth leader is a construction supervisor!) or maybe even come to Woodland and work with our Samoset Ministry. Isn't that just very cool....all from an empty coffee pot!!

Monday, February 7

We're getting closer! They discharged Keith from the hospital yesterday morning, so he was able to watch the Super Bowl on a decent TV and sleep in a comfy bed last night. When we went in this morning we found out several things...first, the HCG was at 2.3, completely in the normal range! that is great news. His platelets were low, so they gave him a transfusion. (By the way, small commercial inserted here...if you are reading this and you are a Woodland member, there will be a blood and platelet drive at Woodland this Sunday. While you can't give directly for Keith, there is no way he could have gone through all of this without people donating, so please do!)

Anyway, the doctor came in and said that she was open to going ahead and releasing Keith if he would go when we got to my mom's house and have bloodwork done at her local hospital, in case he needed more platelets. I said, "That makes me nauseated to think about that. We need to just stay here until you are completely comfortable with him traveling." So, for now we are staying until Wednesday. They will reevaluate on Wednesday morning, and then we will decide if we can leave or if we need to stay another day. Hey, after 50 days, what's another 1 or 2? I just want to be sure he is in good enough health to make the trip!

When he was finished today, they told him he was free to go out to eat if he wanted to, so we went to a restaurant that some friends here at the hotel had told us about. It is called Maxine's Chicken and Waffles, and, Oh My, My...was it ever good! There was a very large African American man doing the cooking, who we later found out was the owner and "Maxine's" grandson. We had fried chicken and fried corn and collard greens and blackeyed peas and cornbread...I tell you, I think Keith's tail was wagging when we left! He shook that big man's hand and said, "That's the best food I've had since I've been here!" Big man said, "God bless you, man...keep the faith!" It was a happy experience!

Tuesday, February 8

We had a really special thing happen this morning. Keith is a member of a group called Metro 2 Music. this is a group of 50 Music Ministers that meet together every year. They are meeting right now in Birmingham, Alabama. This morning they called and asked if they could Skype Keith in to their meeting. It was really cool to see all of those guys. Keith told them a little about our journey here, and then they had a special prayer time for him.

Other than that, our day was uneventful. We packed a little bit this afternoon, and we are really hoping to be on the road tomorrow. I won't be able to update this if we get to travel until we get home, so if you don't hear from me for a few days, just know that we were able to leave.

Right now please just pray for all the counts, for his strength to return, and the side effects (neuropathy and hearing) to lessen.

Sunday, February 13

We are home!! It was quite an eventful journey...last Wednesday they made the decision that he could leave, so we began to pack the car around noon. It was 12 degrees. As I went to get the car to pull it up, I fell on the ice! I couldn't believe I had made it over 50 days negotiating the ice and snow, and then managed to fall during the last hour! I was okay, though, and we finally got on the road.

We stopped for lunch in Louisville, then headed to Lexington, where it began snowing. The weather turned bad really fast, and we were crawling along the interstate. It took us 5 hours to drive 165 miles! We finally gave up and stopped at a hotel just north of Knoxville. We were exhausted by the time we got to the room!

On Thursday we made it to my mom's, and spent Thursday and Friday with her. We got in last night about 7:30 pm, and it is SO good to be home. Keith is feeling well, just tired. We have an appointment with our doctor here tomorrow. I'm sure he'll want a full report on everything Indy!

Tuesday, February 15

Still enjoying sunny Florida! It's hard for me to remember how cold we were!

Keith met with our oncologist here on Monday. He was very pleased with the results. His only disagreement was with the decision not to do a PET scan. He thinks Keith should have one done in April, just to be sure nothing shows up hot. He had bloodwork and his counts are still very low. May have to have a transfusion on Thursday.

I am back on the hamster wheel...lots of work waiting on me! Hopefully I can get caught up and get all of our stuff put back in place this week!

Monday, February 21

Keith's counts are still holding at about the same. Still low, but at least they are not going down. They have made the decision not to do any transfusions yet. Hopefully things will start heading up this week.

But I do have news, and you are really not going to believe this one. I went to my doctor on Thursday for my last "post surgery" checkup. (for those who don't know, I had a hysterectomy in late October). I was supposed to go in January but for obvious reasons had to put it off. When he checked my incision area he got a really weird look, and said…"you have a large hernia. We need to get you in for a CT scan immediately." To which I responded…."What do you do for a large hernia?" He said, "surgery." I sat straight up, looked him square in the eye and said, "Are you kidding me?" Long story short, I had the CT scan on Friday and appointment with the surgeon today, and surgery is scheduled for March 10. It is a large hernia (4" long) that goes right along the inside incision from my surgery. Apparently I was not as well as I thought I was when we went to Indy. Then, I caught a cold in that God-forsaken weather, and my coughing tore it loose.

So…in the never ending saga of the Martins, this is the latest chapter. I will probably have to spend one night in the hospital, but recovery will be relatively quick. Just have to be sure I don't catch any colds afterward.

One thing is for sure...our life is never dull!!

Monday, February 28

Keith went to the office today for what was supposed to be a half day, but he ended up staying until around 2 pm, when he had a doctor's appointment. He was so glad to be back at work. I wish these stubborn cells would start moving so he wouldn't have to be so careful! they are still low. We talked with the Nurse Practitioner from Indiana today, and I think they are going to order him a Neupagin shot for Thursday. Hopefully that will give things a boost.

Monday, March 7

Keith went to the doctor today, and his counts have come up a little. His white count is at 3 (on its way to 10), but red count and platelets are still about the same. He is having a lot of issues with the neuropathy in his feet. The doctor says that it is actually encouraging that it is bothering him so much, as it may be a sign that the nerves are trying to wake up.

He led worship this weekend, and was so glad to be back with the Woodland people. They were very welcoming, as well. He received cheers at every service!

Tuesday, March 15

I apologize for not writing before now. I love all of your gentle chiding emails...and I am so thankful that you worry about me! My surgery was last Thursday, and everything went fine. I had to spend one night in the hospital, but it took me all weekend to truly come out of the anesthesia! I literally slept all day Friday, Saturday and Sunday! I went back to the doctor yesterday and he is very pleased with my progress. don't worry, I am being a very good patient...not lifting anything! I DON'T want to have to go through this again!

Keith counts are still holding at about the same. He is red count is up a little, so he feels stronger, but the white count is still hovering at 3. Dr. Einhorn is keeping a close watch on him. Our oncologist was pleased that Dr. Einhorn has called him twice! Please pray for these counts to recover.

Monday, March 28

Keith and I have both been recovering pretty well. I had my stitches taken out today. I still have a surgical drain that I am really ready to get rid of, and it will hopefully come out next week.

Keith is doing pretty well. His white count is still low, but right now everyone is just waiting and watching. He had a "phone meeting" with Dr. Einhorn today, so I am interested to see what all he had to say about the low white count.

Other than that, life is moving on. My mother has been here visiting this week, which has been very nice. She will fly back to Cleveland tomorrow.

Tuesday, March 29 (personal journal)

I am writing this to keep up with all that I am feeling, and try and keep sane. When we returned from Indiana, I had to have surgery on Thursday, March 10. The following Monday, we found out that Keith's HCG tumor marker had started to rise again. The doctors immediately ordered a PET scan, and the scan showed nothing…no tumors or hot spots. This is good, but yesterday Dr. Einhorn called and told Keith that he felt sure that the rising HCG (from 98 to 179 to 290) indicated microscopic disease in the bloodstream. He wants us to wait until May or June, have a CT scan, then come up there to meet with him. The next step would be additional chemotherapy that are different drugs than Keith has had before. The problem is…there is only a 30% success rate with this.

The thing that freaked me out the most is that this is the last bullet in the treatment gun. If this doesn't work, there is not anything else. Keith pushed him on what that meant…as in how long…and he said it would take 2-3 years before the disease would take his life.

I cried myself to sleep last night, then woke up and stared at the ceiling for 2 hours. It has never really occurred to me that Keith wouldn't come through this. His faith is strong. He is asking God for a miracle and believing that if he has to have the chemo that it will work. I love him so much and can't bear to see him have to go through more treatment.

Right now we are not telling anyone about this. My mother knows, but she is the only one aside from healthcare people. We have decided to wait until we meet with Dr. Einhorn in May to tell anyone. There is no reason, since we don't know anything.

I am realizing that I am in a place of no control. I have to trust and wait. In case you haven't noticed, I'm not so good on the waiting part. I guess the good thing about this right now is that since no one knows, it is a very personal journey. I am seeking God with all my heart. I am asking Him to heal Keith, but I know that He may not. My verse for this last portion of the journey has been Jeremiah 29:11-14:
11 For I know the plans I have for you," declares the LORD, "plans to prosper you and not to harm you, plans to give you hope and a future. 12 Then you will call on me and come and pray to me, and I will listen to you. 13 You will seek me and find me when you seek me with all your heart.

Today I also read the following verse:
Romans 8:24 - *24 For in this hope we were saved. But hope that is seen is no hope at all. Who hopes for what they already have?*

Thursday, May 12 (personal journal)

There have not been a lot of changes since I last wrote, just a lot of plans made and some gut honest talks. I was really, really torn up for several days after the initial talk with Dr. Einhorn, almost to the point that I couldn't even talk about it. Keith and I made a decision that we would not tell anyone about this until after the Indiana appointment, and we would have to fine a way to not make this the absolute focus of our life. There have been several significant things that have happened.

First, just a few days after the Dr. E. conversation, I was in the shower and had another one of my "God moments." It was just like the time in the hospital the first weekend that Keith got sick. It was so real that it almost seemed audible, and I felt God say, "That man has no idea when Keith is going to die." IU was reminded again that while we are so grateful to have such a famous doctor as Keith's doctor…it is only God that knows the number of days that we will be on earth.

Second, I began feverishly doing some research about possible reasons Keith could have a high HCG with no evidence of disease. He could have an antibody called a heterophile antibody that would give a false positive HCG. If the test in Indy show high HCG with no evidence still of disease, I'm going to ask Dr. Einhorn about testing him for it. There have been cases reported but it is very rare.

Finally, I pray every night for God to heal him. I place my hands on him and quietly pray for god's complete healing. We stopped getting the HCG results several weeks ago because thee was nothing we could do about it, and all it did was cause us anxiety. We go back to Indy on May 23-24. Keith has a CT scan on the morning of the 24th followed by an appointment with Dr. Einhorn. I am claiming that the tests will be normal and the scans will be clear. But I know that if God has other plans, we will accept them.

Right after Keith talked with Dr. Einhorn, one of Bethany and Trey's friends from Auburn died of brain cancer. This was a young man 22 years old that left behind a young wife and child. When Keith heard about it he said, "You know, I'm sure that young man would have given anything to have lived to age 52!" I guess we all think the appropriate time to die is around 80 or 90. But I'm not sure we are ever ready or ready to give up the ones we love.

We have been quietly checking on life insurance and other things. General information, but our plan is not to need it for a long time.

Our next few weeks are busy…next week a trip to Disney for my birthday. May 23-24, the trip to Indy. May 29, we drive to Dallas to move Josh back home. He begins a new job here on June 6. Then June 13-18 we are in Hawaii to celebrate our 30th anniversary. July 8 Keith leaves for the Navajo mission trip.

Friday, June 10

What a week! I can't believe I am writing here again, but unfortunately, it means there is news to report on Keith's health. Last Monday he went to the doctor for a routine checkup and some bloodwork. Everything was moving along okay until the doctor noticed his hemoglobin count. I was at 8.2, down from 12.3 three weeks ago. After he found that everything went into a tailspin, as there should be no reason for Keith to be losing blood unless he was bleeding somewhere. He first assumed that Keith had a bleeding ulcer in his stomach. Trying to get him in for tests this week proved to be challenging, but we had to have the tests this week because our 30th anniversary trip to Hawaii was planned for a Monday departure!

After a little while of trying to work everything out, he decided to admit Keith to the hospital. There they could do all the tests that they needed to and give him blood transfusions at the same time. So, they admitted him for what was to be one day on Tuesday. Wednesday morning he was scheduled for the endoscopy. I didn't worry about getting down there before he went for the test, as it is a very routine test. He called me right after the test and said that they were going to do a CT of his lung and he would meet me in the room after the test. When I got to his room, I saw in his little plastic pan that he had been spitting up blood. It scared me to death! Luckily he was back in the room within 30 minutes and said that he had started coughing up blood at about 6 that morning. The CT scan, however looked the same as it had two weeks ago in Indiana...a few places of concern, but nothing major. The endoscopy was clear except they did find blood in his stomach, but couldn't find the source. So, they decided to do a colonoscopy the next day. Prep for that was lovely...he had to drink a gallon of yukky stuff.

So, on Thursday morning he went down for the colonoscopy. While they had him down there, they made the decision to do a boronchiloscopy (sp?) Not sure if that's even the name of it, but it is a scope that goes into your lung. Keith said every orifice in his body has had a scope put in it this week! Because he had both of these done within an hour of each other, his body spiked a fever to fight what it perceived as an invasion. His fever got up to 102 that afternoon and he could not stop shaking. The fever finally broke at 11 pm last night.

Unfortunately, the lung scope revealed the true culprit. They found a small tumor in his left lung and the tumor is bleeding. The cure for bleeding tumors in lungs is radiation. They will give him 10 rounds of low dose radiation beginning on Monday. The goal is to cauterize the tumor to stop the bleeding, which they feel 100% certain that they can do. An additional benefit is that the radiation doctor also believes it will destroy the tumor.

So, instead of going to Hawaii on Monday we will be heading in for yet another cancer treatment. I came home today and canceled everything. I had to fight back tears for some of it, as we have been planning this trip for almost 18 months! We are calling it postponed instead of canceled, and we are hoping to maybe reschedule it in the fall. For those that are wondering, the doctor said Keith will be fine to go on the Navajo mission trip. Of course, I'll be counting on all of you to be praying!!

So, that's the update. The one night in the hospital has turned into 4. Hopefully he will get out tomorrow. They kept him today to be sure and bump up his count, since he is still bleeding. He has pretty much stopped coughing up the blood, but the doc is concerned it could start back.

This is definitely another kink in the rope, but we are okay. Believe it or not, we have seen God's hand in so many ways through this, and have had strong, praying friends gather around us each step of the way. I decided it was time to get the mighty army involved, though! Please pray for the obvious, that the procedure will work and will take care of the tumor. Last weekend at church two of our gals sang the song, "No Matter What" in our services. If you don't know it, it says, "No matter what, I'm going to praise you." I have been singing the song in my head all week, and now I know why. It has been a really rough 48 hours, but God has sustained us, and no matter what, I will praise Him. We love you all.

Saturday, June 11

I promise not to be as long-winded tonight! There is not a lot to tell today. Keith didn't get out of the hospital today, because they wanted to be sure he could hold the blood counts. They also gave him platelets today. As of tonight, his counts were great, and he is really feeling good. It is so funny...he's not hooked up to anything. He has on his pajamas, not the usual hospital gown, and because he feels so good he is giving the nurses fits! He had me bring his robe to the hospital because the doctor wanted him to do some walking. The first time he went out the nurses started calling him Hugh Hefner! For those of you that knew his dad...he's got a lot of Alto Martin in him! Anyway, we feel certain unless something really weird happens tonight that he will come home tomorrow.

I have received lots of emails and calls and texts today, and the thing I want you all to know is that we are fine. Not some kind of "we are in denial" fine, but really okay. It stinks that we had to cancel the vacation, but I can't imagine being in the middle of Maui and having all of this happen. We started today looking at possible days to reschedule.

I don't know what is ahead, but we will take it as it comes. For now, Keith is planning on being back in the office on Tuesday, and we will work this current wrinkle into our lives. This disease is NOT in control. The God we serve controls our future, and we trust Him with it.

Tuesday, June 14

So sorry I haven't updated before now. Yesterday was busy, busy! We went to the oncologist yesterday morning, where Keith got a dose of chemo to make the tumor sensitive to the radiation. After that we headed to the Radiation office where they got Keith prepped and ready to start the radiation today. He will go in about 4 pm today.

The bleeding in the lung has cause him to have shortness of breath, just from standing up and walking across the room. The doctor thinks that will get better after they stop the bleeding. The only bad thing from yesterday is that they gave him steroids with the chemo to limit side effects. That makes it very difficult for him to sleep. Last night he was up and going strong at 1 am, then up and working again around 5:30 this morning. Hopefully he will sleep better tonight.

On a lighter note, we rescheduled the trip for the end of October. Looks like everything they are doing to him should be complete by then. So, back to planning, which most of you know has been my escape during the past 2 years!!

Wednesday, June 15

Keith has been through 2 days of radiation, and so far he likes it a whole lot better than chemo! I know every treatment is different, but for him the radiation is much better! He is still very short of breath, and I think we will probably find tomorrow that his blood counts are low. He is really tired, and his blood pressure is low. We sort of anticipate a transfusion tomorrow. All of that is to be expected with that pesky bleeding in the lung! The radiation oncologist feels certain it will stop the bleeding, but it may not stop until the end of next week.

We had a cool thing happen this week. When we were in the doctors office, one of the women that works there came up to me and asked if she could talk to me. She looked near tears, and when she started to talk, she started to cry, and asked if I would mind going into her office to talk. When we sat down she said she had a friend that knew Keith, and told her that she could trust us. She said she knew we were followers of Christ, and that she is, too. To protect her confidence, I am not going to tell the story of what we talked about, but we had a great talk and I was able to point her to some help and some resources that I think will be beneficial. As well as offer my prayer support. She apologized for bothering me, and I said, "Are you kidding? It is this sort of thing that makes all of "this" (cancer stuff) make sense." One thing I am learning about the purposes of God is that He will move people in and out of our lives to accomplish His purposes. I know I couldn't have had that encounter with that sweet woman if I were in Hawaii. It does help to realize that He is still working. The entire story brought tears to Keith's eyes. I really think what meant the most to him was that the woman's friend had told her that she could trust us.

Then, when we got to the radiation place, the tech was asking Keith all sorts of questions about our church and the services. He shared with Keith about some struggles he is having in his family. Keith gave him a card, and he is supposed to watch our services this weekend online. Please pray for both of these. And continue to pray that God will use us as we travel this road.

Please continue to pray for him, that the radiation will stop the bleeding quickly. There will be more things to think about after that, but that is the most pressing thing.

Bethany came home for the weekend tonight. It will be so great to have both of the kids home for Father's Day.

Thursday, June 16

Sure enough, today brought the news that Keith will need a blood transfusion. He's had so many to this point that it really is not a big deal, and I am really hoping it will make him feel better. They got everything set up today and he will get the transfusion tomorrow morning.

He really feels crummy. He has almost flu-like symptoms: fever, sometimes chills, aches and pains, and extreme fatigue. They really believe it is a combination of the chemo, the radiation, and the lung bleeding. They are not that concerned about the fever, as long as it continues to come right down with Tylenol. It is apparently part of the side effects of all that is going on with him. Apparently as the radiation and the chemo attacks the tumor it can cause fever. Fine with me as long as something is being attacked. The fever, however, is part of what makes him feel so awful.

I don't think he is going to try and lead worship this weekend. Roger was already scheduled to fill in for him because...remember...we are supposed to be in Hawaii!! If the transfusion gives him a big boost, he may try and go in to help with the service.

I hit a rough patch today. I really can not believe we are back at this place again. I sat down and had a good cry, and I feel better. Each time the "cure" has proven to be false, I have had a good cry, and so far this time I hadn't had it and I needed it. Now I'm better, except for that dull headache you have after a good cry!!

Saturday, June 18

Keith had the transfusion yesterday and it really seemed to help. He had a lot more energy last night, and it may be my imagination, but it seems like he is not quite as winded. He is still a long way from normal, but maybe everything is coming together to do what they hoped it would. Please continue to pray, as next week he has to do it all over again (chemo on Monday and radiation on Monday-Friday).

He decided not to try to do anything with the services this weekend. The good thing about having the vacation in place is that we were supposed to be gone this weekend and next, so people are already in place to help out. We are SO thankful for that!

Monday, June 20

Today is our 30th anniversary!! Woo hoo!! We spent the day in the usual routine...oncologist's office and then to radiation. They decided not to give him the chemo today, since his platelets were low (47,000). The drug causes them to drop, so they want him to recover some before they give him more. The great thing is that he didn't have to have the steroids and chemo on our anniversary! They are planning to give it to him on Thursday, which may zap him for the weekend, but that will be his last dose as far as the "radiation chemo." He will have the radiation everyday this week, with the final visit next Monday.

Good news in that he is definitely not as winded. He still coughs up a little blood, so we are not out of the woods yet, but it is definitely better. He felt better today and tonight than he has in a long time. I surely hope it holds! He is planning on going in to the office tomorrow. He's so ready to get back to a little bit of normalcy!

We waited until last minute to make any anniversary plans, as we were not sure if he would be up to it. You really hate to spend $50 on a steak that he can't eat! We ended up at the Riverside Reef Grille in Palmetto. It is a lovely place right on the water. It is a marina, so it is surrounded by beautiful boats. Of course, when we got there I realized that the batteries in my camera were dead! I couldn't believe we were going to have our 30th anniversary with no photos! Then...the photo superman saved the day! Les Urbanski and his daughter were there for a date night, and for those of you who don't know him, Les is an avid photographer, and of course had his camera with him. Let's just say that our evening was adequately documented!! He even made us feed each other dessert so he could get a photo! Thank you again, Les!

Wednesday, June 22

Keith has continued to get stronger, so we are pretty sure that the treatment is doing what they had hoped. He is scheduled to go in tomorrow for blood work and to possibly get the chemo. He is really feeling back to normal, so I am hoping that the chemo doesn't make him sick. Last time his biggest issue was with the steroids that he has to take.

Still not sure if he will lead worship this weekend. Roger is on standby, so I guess it will all depend on how he is feeling after the treatments tomorrow.

Please continue to pray. Keith really wants to be able to go on the Navajo mission trip scheduled for July 8-16. Please pray that his health will improve so he can go, and that we will make the wise decision as to whether or not he should go.

Monday, June 27

Keith had his last radiation treatment today. The doctor was very pleased with his progress, and was especially pleased that he was able to lead worship last weekend. He feels like that gave his lungs a good workout, and he was pleased that it didn't cause any setbacks.

Our next benchmark will be the scans on July 5. We really have no idea what to expect. We assume that the lung spots will show up hot, but they may not even be there any more from the radiation! That would be fine with us. Please be praying about that. We should have the results on the 6th or 7th.

Don't panic if I don't write here until then. Our life has moved back to normal. Keith is back in the office and is working feverishly to prepare for the Navajo mission trip. I promise to update as soon as we have any news. Keep him on your prayer list.

Monday, June 27 (personal journal)

Lots of things have happened since I last wrote…bleeding tumor in the lung, canceled Hawaii trip, radiation. Even a "dear John" letter from Dr. Einhorn, proclaiming that there is nothing else he can do for Keith. (nothing like getting the news of a terminal illness in a letter…with your name spelled wrong!) More detail later, but I had to share what I found tonight through a rather odd series of events.

I have read this passage hundreds of times throughout my life, but I stumbled across it in a rather unique way tonight. Even though I could quote most of it, this passage really spoke to me tonight. Especially the "hope that is seen is no hope at all." God is working in our lives, I know that.

[24] But hope that is seen is no hope at all. Who hopes for what they already have? [25] But if we hope for what we do not yet have, we wait for it patiently.

[26] In the same way, the Spirit helps us in our weakness. We do not know what we ought to pray for, but the Spirit himself intercedes for us through wordless groans. [27] And he who searches our hearts knows the mind of the Spirit, because the Spirit intercedes for God's people in accordance with the will of God.

[28] And we know that in all things God works for the good of those who love him, who have been called according to his purpose. [29] For those God foreknew he also predestined to be

conformed to the image of his Son, that he might be the firstborn
among many brothers and sisters. 30 And those he predestined, he
also called; those he called, he also justified; those he justified, he
also glorified.

31 What, then, shall we say in response to these things? If God is
for us, who can be against us? 32 He who did not spare his own
Son, but gave him up for us all—how will he not also, along with
him, graciously give us all things? 33 Who will bring any charge
against those whom God has chosen? It is God who justifies. 34
Who then is the one who condemns? No one. Christ Jesus who
died—more than that, who was raised to life—is at the right hand
of God and is also interceding for us. 35 Who shall separate us
from the love of Christ? Shall trouble or hardship or persecution
or famine or nakedness or danger or sword? 36 As it is written:

> "For your sake we face death all day long;
> we are considered as sheep to be slaughtered."

37 No, in all these things we are more than conquerors through
him who loved us. 38 For I am convinced that neither death nor
life, neither angels nor demons, neither the present nor the future,
nor any powers, 39 neither height nor depth, nor anything else in
all creation, will be able to separate us from the love of God that
is in Christ Jesus our Lord

We have seen time after time the past few weeks God using what seems to be devastating news and circumstances to bring people closer to him and to work in their lives. God is trustworthy…we are trusting.

Tuesday, July 5

Keith sort hit bottom yesterday...very tired and just rough feeling. He went in today for the PET scan and bloodwork, and while he was waiting on the PET scan he started getting messages that the nurse wanted to see him when he was finished. Come to find out, his red blood count was at 6.2! They immediately sent over to the hospital to get a blood transfusion, which took all day. He just took his computer and did a bunch of work while he was there.

I went back to pick him up around 6:30 and we went down to the beach and had dinner at one of our favorite places where you eat right on the sand! It was wonderful, and the sunset was beautiful. Just what we needed after a stress-filled day!

We will meet with the doctor tomorrow to see if we can figure out what is going on inside of him. Please pray.

Thursday, July 7

I am so sorry I didn't get to write yesterday. Our power went out at 8 pm last night and we just went to bed. Also, if any of you tried to call our house, the phones weren't working due to the lack of power. We are out the door this morning headed to a doctor's appointment, so my time is limited. I promise more later.

The scan did confirm that the cancer has returned, and that there is bleeding in his lung again. He is going in this morning for another transfusion, and will start chemo on Monday. This chemo consists of different drugs to hopefully halt the progress of this monster.

As you can tell, we need your prayers desperately. I will write more later.

Thursday, July 7 (personal journal)

This has been a really tough week. The scans on Tuesday revealed that Keith has many cancer spots all over him. They are not sure what this cancer is, but it appears to be very aggressive. They did a brain scan yesterday and the results of that revealed today that he has cancer spots on his brain and on his skull. The harsh reality from all of this is that Keith has about a month to live.

I have cried an awful lot in the past 24 hours, and have evaluated a lot. I am so thankful for the 2 years that God gave us after the diagnosis. We crammed a lot of living and loving into those 2 years and for that I will always be thankful. Don't get me wrong…I am devastated and would give anything if I could hold on to him for a few more years, but the reality is that I would never be ready for this to happen.

So, we are entering a very difficult time, these last days. I am asking God for peace and mercy, and begging that Keith will not have to suffer. I wish it was me. Or even better, I wish we could go together.

Friday, July 8 (personal journal)

The past 24 hours have been a whirlwind. There is a chance that Keith's health will deteriorate rapidly, so he has been busy as a beaver trying to do all the preparations. One of my favorites is this email that he sent to Eric Botts, a funeral director in Tennessee that will help oversee Keith's funeral:

Eric,

I have bad news from today's appointment that nobody knows about yet: my caner has moved to multiple parts of my body and now the brain. It is terminal and untreatable. I only have 4 weeks left to live and of that, only 1-2 weeks of quality of life. So I need to make some decisions ***fast.***

Funeral Home Details:

Things I need to secure price for (or can you negotiate for us) are: picking up body, embalming body and preparing body, receiving casket from you, transportation to and from church for both visitation and burial, overseeing both those events, newspaper notices, transportation of body to Greenwood Cemetery in Montgomery, AL where I have a plot. I guess I/we need to negotiate with Greenwood the prep of plot, vault, and actual burial

Casket:

I guess you don't test drive these things, but assume you will email me some options (low end will be fine). I want decide this as soon as possible. Also, I want to decide on all of those little extras that seem to add up.

Headstone:

This is the one thing I have not thought of till now. Can you help us with this? If yes, I want to secure that price and ordering process, then firm up a price with Greenwood to install it.

What have I forgotten? Just email both LeeAnn and I your thoughts and ideas, or feel free to call us at the house at any time.

I can't thank you enough for this and want you to know from my heart what a privilege it has been to mentor and walk beside your brother. He is a special man of the Lord.

Keith Martin

That is so typically Keith…to go ahead and organize his funeral and all of the arrangements. He has also already planned the service!

Bethany came in last night, so it is good to have both children here. Trey, Bethany's boyfriend is flying in today, and Paul and Mariann are coming on Wednesday. We decided to try and visit with a lot of folks now, in case his health deteriorates suddenly, which they think it could do. We also have an appointment today with an estate attorney to be sure our will is in order.

This is so surreal. Keith looks fine and acts fine, except for being a little winded. Yet this monster is destroying his body from the inside.

We woke up early this morning and snuggled and laughed. I asked Keith if he was scared and he said, "No. The only thing I am nervous about is the actual dying process. I just don't want to linger." Trusting God for today.

Saturday, July 9 (personal journal)

We have accomplished a lot in the past 48 hours. Keith has been busy writing emails and making lists, and I have been trying to tell the people that need to know first. That's a really tough thing, as of course, the news hits them like a ton of bricks! I have cried several times already today.

We met with the estate attorney yesterday to be sure that all is in order with our will and living will and power of attorney and stuff. I think everything is pretty much taken care of. He still wants to talk with a local funeral home, so I guess we will do that on Monday. We will also start with hospice on Monday.

Yesterday at Florida Cancer, Keith had an opportunity to talk with several of the nurses, and to encourage them in their faith.

We were aware of other people around, but really didn't think about it. Yesterday afternoon Keith received the following email:

Keith,

I was at Florida Cancer Specialists today and Denise and Carly told me you had received "bad news". I wanted you to know that marveled at your composure, that you were encouraging them, that you had peace in the midst of this. I've prayed for, counseled and encouraged these ladies for the last two years and have seen God doing remarkable things in their lives. Thank you for being a part of that.

Thank you also for the time we shared in the chemo room. It was quite an encouragement and blessing to me. I have prayed for you often and will continue to do so.

My time at FCS is coming to an end. Right now we are just checking my counts monthly to be sure but my platelette count has stabilized in the normal range. No more bleeding, no more anemia - no more treatments. God did not grant me the miraculous healing we sought, but He did miraculously provide for my healing and in the process gave me the opportunity to testify to His greatness, provide encouragement and participate in His work as He restored 2 marriages and brought 2 of His children back home. It wasn't fun, but it was so worth it.

I have seen God glorified in you at FCS and pray that He will enable you to know the fullness of your participation in His ministry there. Peace and Blessings

Today we are doing fun stuff…floating in the pool, remembering fun stories, and laughing a lot. At times it seems surreal. Keith looks so normal. I can't imagine what lies ahead for us. I am praying for God's mercy.

He held me last night in bed as I cried. Yesterday Josh and I took some people to the airport to leave on the mission trip. Being at the airport made me cry. We have gone on so many fun trips from there. I definitely have really rough times, but I am determined to enjoy the last weeks that we have together.

Sunday, July 10 (personal journal)

Keith is getting weaker. It is absolutely amazing to me that a week ago he led worship in both services, and then went to a Rays game. AND that we didn't know any of this was coming. I really can't imagine him being able to continue like this a long time. He gets so winded just moving around the house.

Hospice is coming tomorrow, and we are telling the staff and the world tomorrow. I am dreading the week. Praying for God to be our sustainer.

Monday, July 11

The time has come for me to update you on what is going on in our lives. You have been so faithful to pray for us through all this journey.

This past week after several scans, including a brain scan, it was determined that the cancer has spread all over Keith's body, and is also on the surface of his brain and on his skull.

The result of this is that there are no more treatments left to do, and they are only predicting that Keith will live another few weeks.

We were told back in March that the cancer was probably not going to be cured, and at that time the doctors thought he had up to 2 years. However, this latest discovery has moved the timeline up drastically. It helped us to take the initial blow back then and gave us time to really get our affairs in order.

Up until today, Keith has really felt good...and has been a busy bee planning his funeral, talking with funeral directors...doing all the typical Keith organized things! I have to tell you that God's peace has surrounded us every step of the way. Week before last especially I felt closer to God than I have in my entire life. Sometime I will tell you all about that. I knew He was preparing me for something, and now I know it was this devastating news.

For now, please just pray for us. We are praying for God's grace and mercy. We are praying that Keith's mind will stay clear until the end.

Bethany and Josh are both here now. Bethany's boyfriend is here, and Josh's girlfriend comes in next Sunday. Keith really wants some quality time with them. We are trying to guard the time we have left to focus on our family and closest friends. Please do not try and come by and visit. Just send emails and notes and we will get them.

He is the absolute love of my life, and it is killing me to see him go through all of this, but I know God is honoring his faithful service, and even now is using him and his story to reach many people.

I promise to update this page daily, so you can check in on how he is doing and anything specific that I need for you to pray about. We met with hospice this morning, and they are taking over his care and providing us with things that will help.

He went in for bloodwork today and will have a blood transfusion tomorrow. These are palliative now, with the goal being to give him energy to help get through the things he wants to accomplish over the next few weeks. Please pray to that end, that it will help him.

I love you all and thank you again for your friendship, notes and prayers. We are really going to need them over the next few weeks.

Tuesday, July 12

Today was spent for the most part at Blake hospital where Keith got a blood transfusion. We met with Hospice yesterday and they approved for him to have an additional couple of transfusions as needed to give him a little more quality of life. Last night was really rough...he had trouble sleeping, and was absolutely wiped out this morning. He couldn't even get out of bed without assistance, and then had to go to the car in shifts...first to the table, catch his breath, then to the car. However, when we got to the hospital and put the oxygen on him, he immediately felt better. He perked up and regained some color in his face. That was even before he got the blood!

We contacted Hospice this afternoon, and they are having oxygen delivered to us this evening, and hopefully that will help him rest better tonight.

The blood and platelet transfusion took 6 hours, and we spent a good portion of that time reading the over 300 emails and 175 Facebook posts that Keith had. I wanted to be sure that you knew that we read every one of them. His vision has started to be affected, so he has trouble reading the computer screen, so I read them all to him. While we can't respond to all of them, I wanted you to know how very much we enjoyed hearing from all of you. He loved all the emails, but especially enjoyed the ones with funny memories. In some ways it was gut wrenching, but more than that it was exhaustingly wonderful.

Keith is a blessed man indeed to be able to hear all of these things before he dies. His ministry really has touched a whole lot of lives. It was really inspiring to read of the young ministers that he mentored that now have congregations and ministries of their own. Such a legacy.

This afternoon I had to talk with the funeral directors and look at caskets...the icky reality of what is happening. I want to get it all done, though, so it can be set aside and we can just enjoy him knowing all the plans are made.

Keith is definitely getting weaker. I created a page on this site that I thought you might enjoy. It is the worship set from the last time Keith led worship on July 3. It is mind-blowing that it was just 9 days ago. He is so much weaker now. We certainly had no idea at the time that it would be the last time he would lead worship. Now he is so weak he has difficulty even sitting on the side of the bed.

There has also been a website created, that has proclaimed July 18 as a prayer day for him. We are truly blessed and overwhelmed by the outpouring, and again, I am so grateful that Keith is still here and is able to read all the things you have written. You will never know how much you all mean to us.

Wednesday, July 13

The oxygen came last night, and it really seemed to help Keith breathe better. He had some problems sleeping, but his breathing was a little better. He is definitely a lot weaker today. He gets so winded even doing the slightest things. We made the decision to get a hospital bed to hopefully help him to sleep by elevating his head.

We had to make some "final" decisions today. It has been a rough one...choosing a casket (I printed out the photos that the director sent, and Keith picked the one he wanted). Stinky thing to have to do. THEN we had a hospital bed moved into our bedroom. Stinky thing #2. The reality of all of this is looming. I really wish I could wake up from this bad dream.

Paul and Mariann Strozier came in today for a few days from Ohio. They are some of our best friends, and Paul is a pastor to Keith (to both of us). We cried together, laughed, and then cried some more, and then laughed some more. It did Keith a lot of good to have some time to talk with Paul. We are so glad they are here.

Keith is having some problems with his vision, so I will ask that you not send anymore emails to his address. If you want to send an email to him, send it to my address, and I will print it out and read it to him. He still really enjoys hearing from everyone. After reading an especially touching email last night (thank you, Todd Bell), Keith said, "I don't want to go." I said, "So, don't." He said, "I have to, everybody has already said all of these nice things about me!" I said, "No, I think it would be good for God to do a miraculous healing so all of these people could tell all of their friends what God did!" That would be SOOO cool!!!

We are so blessed to have our kids here. They are doing a good bit of "parenting their parents," and doing a good job of it! So proud of them.

Without a doubt, this is the hardest thing I have ever done. Please continue to pray.

Thursday, July 14

Keith is getting weaker by the day (almost by the hour). It is tearing me apart, but it is such an honor to be able to take care of him. And he always thanks me and apologizes when he thinks he has been a bother. I have been such a blessed woman to be able to walk with him for these 30 years.

Paul and Mariann have been such a blessing to us already. Mariann has been cleaning and washing clothes, and Paul has helped me so much taking care of Keith. He and Keith came up with a playlist today for Keith's ipod of all of Keith's favorite songs so he could have them playing as he gets weaker. Paul is absolutely his best friend, and they have had many good talks and have cried many tears together.

It has been interesting to hear how it seems God is waking people up at night in all different areas to pray for us. I really believe there is a 24 hour prayer chain that is ordained by God. It's that whole thing of the Spirit interceding for us when we don't know how to pray. I keep hearing God say, "Trust me," and I do.

Keith has received now over 700 emails. The stories and memories have been wonderful. I am so amazed at the number of young ministers that he mentored through the years that now have their own churches and recall how much he invested in their lives.

Several of you have commented on my allowing you into our lives at this pivotal time. My desire is to help you all understand, dear ones, that when you reach this point in your life that God will surround you just as he has us. It is my hope that you will realize that whatever you are facing he has promised to be with you. He will strengthen you and he will comfort you as He is doing us now. This is not easy, but Keith's reward is just around the bend. My greatest sadness is that I can't go with him.

Friday, July 15 – 4 am

Early this morning, my sweet Keith was ushered into the presence of Jesus. It happened faster than we had expected, but God was merciful. Yesterday evening, he was struggling so much to breathe. While he was trying to sleep, I told God, "Please go ahead and take him. He's fought so hard." I found out later that Paul had actually prayed the same thing when he was sitting with Keith. So, at 1:06 this morning that is what happened. Josh, Bethany and I were all with him. I am heartbroken but thankful, as he was really beginning to suffer.

As I sat by him and looked at his worn out earthly shell, I was in awe to know that he is now in the presence of Jesus. And without a doubt he is hearing the words, "Well done, good and faithful servant."

As I close I want to leave you with this passage of scripture:

Revelation 22:1-4
1 *Then the angel showed me the river of the water of life, as clear*
as crystal, flowing from the throne of God and of the Lamb 2
down the middle of the great street of the city. On each side of the
river stood the tree of life, bearing twelve crops of fruit, yielding
its fruit every month. And the leaves of the tree are for the
healing of the nations. 3 *No longer will there be any curse. The*
throne of God and of the Lamb will be in the city, and his
servants will serve him. 4 *They will see his face, and his name*
will be on their foreheads. 5 *There will be no more night. They*
will not need the light of a lamp or the light of the sun, for the
Lord God will give them light. And they will reign for ever and
ever.

I miss him desperately already, but I am very envious of all he is experiencing right now. Thank you, dear friends for the way you poured out your love on him this past week.

Friday, July 15 - 8 pm

It's difficult to believe that I wrote that last post just this morning. Today has been very long. It has been good, though as we have remembered so many good times. I wanted to take a moment this evening to be sure you were all aware of the plans for Keith's services. Here is the obituary:

Alan Keith Martin, 53, of Bradenton, FL joined the worship gathering in heaven on Friday July 15. Keith was born May 5, 1958 in Montgomery, AL. He was preceded in death by parents Alto Martin and Lois Price Martin. He was married to the former LeeAnn Lofty on June 20, 1981 and they have two children, Joshua and Bethany, both of Bradenton. Keith served for over 31 years as a Worship Pastor for churches in Texas, Oklahoma, Alabama, Indiana and, for the past six years, at Woodland – The Community Church in Bradenton. Keith was a faithful follower of Jesus Christ who led others through his own authentic heart for worship. His legacy consists of his love for Christ, family, and friends, his mentorship of over fifty persons currently in ministry, and thousands of worshipers around the world. Arrangements are under the care of Snow's Funeral Ministry (352) 438-0007. Family visitation will be held Thursday, July 21 from 6:00-9:00 p.m. and the worship celebration will be Friday, July 22 at 11:00 a.m., both at Woodland, 9607 State Road 70, E., Bradenton, FL. The worship service will be streamed via www.woodlandlive.com. A graveside service will be held Saturday, July 23 at 11:00 a.m. at Greenwood Cemetery in Montgomery, AL. Rev. Tim Passmore of Bradenton and Rev. Paul Strozier of Columbus, OH will co-officiate. Flowers may be sent to Woodland Church and donations may be made to The Navajo Mission Fund, c/o Woodland or online at www.gowoodland.com. Keith finished strong.

Just a note about the service: Many of you Valleydale members have mentioned remembering Keith singing the song, " Heaven."

I wanted to let you know that we will be playing the recording of him singing that in the service on Friday. I can think of no greater thing than to hear Keith's beautiful voice singing that song...and knowing that he is there.

I am exhausted, as I didn't sleep at all last night. I am about to take some sleeping aides and crash. Please pray for rest for all of us.

Saturday, July 16

We all slept well last night and today has been a quiet day.

For today's posting, I wanted to share with you a blog posting that a pastor from Mobile wrote about Keith last week. It was written by Brett Burleson. He is the pastor of Dayspring Church in Mobile, Alabama. He was one of our "kids" when we were at First Baptist North Mobile. He very eloquently stated how Keith spent his time investing in all of these young men and women that he liked to call his "Row of Honor." In the final arrangement document that Keith wrote out for us to use, here is what he wrote about all of these young ministers:

The highest honor I've had in life is the mentoring of these young men and women. I don't know if or how much I've impacted their lives, but I sure did enjoy doing it. When I stand before the Lord, I truly believe He's not going to ask about the big productions I did or say "Put Keith in the Tide Pride section because his choir was over a 100", but He's going to ask each one of us "Who did you leave in your place to carry on the work of the kingdom?"

Here is what Brett wrote:

Nostalgia

"Remember your leaders, who spoke the word of God to you. Consider the outcome of their way of life and imitate their faith." (Hebrews 13:7)

I've been stricken with nostalgia today. I absolutely can't shake it. And I know why. A good friend of mine appears to be living his final days on this earth. He has been fighting cancer for some time now, and the doctors are saying his body won't last much longer.

I guess I need to define what I mean by "good friend," because I (like many) tend to use the term loosely. Some refer to anyone on their Facebook roster as a good friend. For others, they narrow a good friend down to someone they spend time with regularly. For others, a good friend is simply someone they want people to think they are actually friends with. In those respects I guess I've got a lot of good friends. Maybe hundreds. But I only have a few friends like this person. Literally only a few.

His name is Keith Martin.

When I became a Christian, Keith was one of the pastors at my church. He was responsible for all the praise, music, etc. He was about thirty years old at the time and was very good at what he did. A real innovator in his field. But his skill and innovation are not why he is so special to me. I spent significant time with Keith in all four of my college years. Two of those college years I worked with him (I was an intern at the church). The other two college years I was involved in a traveling ministry team that Keith directed. Outside of family, I spent more time with Keith than any other adult.

And I watched him. Oftentimes very closely.

During those years Keith talked with me. He read the Bible to me. He made me do things (like sing in church and go on mission trips). He encouraged me to become a pastor, and also encouraged me to marry April. He let me see him do things well. And he even let me see him lose his cool. He saw something in me that I, quite frankly, didn't see. And he told me so. Keith mentored me and showed me what a good husband, father, minister, and man looks like. And he did a superb job of it.

Keith Martin's life is a reminder that what you do matters, and that the life you live has residual effects. I (like literally dozens of my hometown peers) followed in Keith's footsteps of vocational ministry. Were it not for him, we probably would never have taken that path (or at least would have had no clue of what to actually do on that path).

Thank you, Keith. You are special. A rare breed. I don't know why God would see fit to allow a guy like you to be in my life during those extremely formative years. But He did. And I'm eternally grateful.

Should I ever have the good fortune of having a young pastor write a blog like this about me one day, much of the credit should go to you.

I love you, my good friend. Always will.

Tuesday, July 19

So thankful for all the many friends, notes, for the food, and the love that we feel from all of you during this difficult week. I created the program for the service today and it is going to be really great...of course it is....Keith Martin planned it all! I hope you will all be able to join us or watch online.

Wednesday, July 20

The past few days have been a time of sweet respite with our family...I know tomorrow will begin an emotional whirlwind and I really covet your prayers. I am overwhelmed with all the many, many people that Keith's life touched. We are expecting big crowds here at the service and in Montgomery. Please pray for peace in the midst of all the chaos. I love you all.

Monday, July 25

The services last week and over the weekend were so wonderful. There were stories and laughter and tears...Keith would have loved every moment of it. The service on Friday was one he planned, even down to the inclusion of the Tithe Rap. He said, "You all are going to need a little laughter by this time of the service!" It was so nice to reconnect with so many friends on Saturday in Montgomery. Even though many of them I only got to hug, it still meant so much that everyone made the journey to be there with us.

The online service was viewed by over 350 separate log ins in 33 states. I should have the video of the service available soon for those who were unable to view it. I will also put together a page of videos of Keith that we have archived on our church site for you to watch.

Today has been quiet. I am back working again. Josh has been home today, and Bethany will be coming back in this evening. Still can't believe we are living all of this, but God is faithfully showing things along the way.

Last night I received a sweet message from a young woman who lost her father suddenly last week. Her father was only 51 years old and was a member of the church we served at in Mobile. David sang in the choir and in ensembles with Keith, but we had never met his daughter. Apparently, several weeks ago David showed this blog to his daughter. She commented on marveling at my ability to still trust God even though our circumstances were so difficult. David died of a heart attack last Wednesday. She spoke of remembering the things I had written. She wrote, "You have set an example that I am trying to follow and thru your loss, you used it as a way to honor the Lord. I just want to thank you for allowing me and others to enter your world and see how God can move." What a precious gift from God this note was. What a huge encouragement! Please pray for the Strong family as they are moving through this most difficult time.

Wednesday, July 27

We are doing okay. As those of you who have been through this know, the grief hits me at strange times, and usually when I am not expecting it. It's okay, though, I just cry a little while and move on. One of my friends brought me a gift bag full of all different sizes of Kleenex and a bunch of chocolate. That definitely helps!

Tuesday, August 2

Thank you so much for all the many, many cards, notes, emails, and Facebook messages that all of you have sent to us. We feel your love, but most of all, we know you are praying for us.

I am amazed at how God is moving people into my life to help with some of the biggest things that I have to see about, and how He is there for comfort during those quiet times of overwhelming grief. I still have a really hard time believing that Keith is not here with us. It still seems like every afternoon he should come through the front door, bigger than life, laughing and playing with the dog. It's real, but I am constantly reminded that God is near me and oftentimes carrying me. Throughout this entire journey we have claimed Jeremiah 29:11-13, and I continue to claim it: *"[11] For I know the plans I have for you," declares the LORD, "plans to prosper you and not to harm you, plans to give you hope and a future. [12] Then you will call on me and come and pray to me, and I will listen to you. [13] You will seek me and find me when you seek me with all your heart."*

Yesterday I had 4 different people tell me of ways they were inspired to minister because of Keith's life. A friend told me that her husband had begun to teach a Bible study at a youth home because of Keith's influence. Another mentioned that her husband shared with an Air Conditioning Repairman that came to their home. She said that Keith's life had inspired him to boldness. Another friend talked about hearing a widow question whether or not her husband's life had mattered. My friend said to me, "I want to be sure you know, Keith's life mattered." Finally, I got an email that I wanted to share with you from a couple in our church:

I just wanted you to know what happened to us last Sunday. We counted money after the last service and were the last ones out of church about 130pm. A car drove up with 3 men in it. They were asking for the pastor. They said they were looking for food and all the food banks were closed. The one man said he was taking chemo with the pastor a year and a half ago. The man said the pastor told him if he ever needed anything to come to this church. The church was all locked up so we took them to SweetBay to buy groceries. I couldn't help but think that Keith is still ministering to people we never imagined. The man said Keith told him to "be strong" and "never give up". He said he was taking care of 3 of his nieces and nephews.
What an opportunity it was for us to minister in Keith's name.

So, with all of these stories, how can I be sad? I rejoice that Keith's ministry and legacy is moving forward in the lives of all of these people. And I have to tell you, my faith in God is broad enough to allow for the possibility that all of this happened to

Keith so that Joe would go to teach those young people, and one of them would come to Christ and continue the work. I know God links together all of us for His purpose, and I am continuously amazed at how deep and broad the influence is. I also know that viewing things with Kingdom eyes helps us see things that are truly profound.

Keith's life did matter. So does yours. And mine. We better get busy.

To quote Keith Martin: "Finish Strong!"

Final words from Keith

On the day that he found out he had only a few weeks to live, Keith sent the following email to our pastor. I thought it appropriate to share it with you as his parting words.

If you were to ask me what the three most important statements that sum up my theme in ministry it would be these:

1 – My calling is to ministry, not to music. While music and worship gets you a church position (training, talent, skill) it is your ministry skills that enable you to touch the people. Ministry is people, not programs. God is not impressed with how big our choir and programs are. God is only interested in changed lives. Every minister will find out one day that our people don't care about our perceived expertise, they just want to know that you care and that you'll be there when needed. A short thank you encouragement email, 2 minute phone call, 5 minute visit in the hospital – that's what they need. Every week, don't just teach them musically, but invest in them spiritually. Let them see the transparency of your life.

2 - I am totally convinced that the only thing that matters in life in the time we have invested in other people's lives. God is not going to ask us in heaven about any of our great accomplishments, but ask us 2 things: (1) how many lives did you allow me to use you as a vessel to change and (2) who did you leave in your place to carry on the kingdom's work?

3 – My kids have heard this one a hundred times in their life: very few people remember how you started, whether it be a job, task, team, relationship, BUT everyone will remember how you finish. FINISH STRONG. When one of my children started a season or project and half way though they got tired, they would get this speech. Think about pastors leaving the ministry, spouses leaving their marriages, people leaving jobs, students quitting teams. In every case I guarantee you that no one

remembers how they started or cared about the so called "great things" they did, but all remember that they quit, left, and tore up others along their way. Don't do it – Finish Strong. I'm very grateful for how I have finished: (1) stayed true to my calling: started 31 years ago in church ministry and finished there, (2) stayed faithful to LeeAnn for 30 years of marriage. I never once cheated on her or flirted elsewhere – I stayed true to her, (3) stayed true to my Lord. I never got drunk, smoked, did drugs, or viewed porn – I did the best I could to keep my mind and life clean so God could use me in every way.

In closing, I have often referred to Laura Story and her statement to our church when she was here in 2008. She shared that she felt that God sends extra trials to his church leaders in order for our people to witness us going through them and how we handle them. I remember flinching when I heard that, yet knowing it was true. As I walked this cancer journey, I have often shared that it is not about me, but how God will use me and this cruel disease to help, encourage, and touch other lives. May it challenge others to do the same – touch lives!

End Notes

[1] Gaither, William J., *These are They*, (1980 William J. Gaither, Inc. ARR UBP of Gaither Copyright Management)

[2] Redmon, Matt., *Blessed Be Your Name*, 2002 Thankyou Music (Admin. by EMI Christian Music Publishing)

[3] Gaither, William J., *It is Finished* (1976 William J. Gaither, Inc. ARR UBP of Gaither Copyright Management)

www.ingramcontent.com/pod-product-compliance
Lightning Source LLC
Chambersburg PA
CBHW030004290326
41934CB00005B/224
9780982612729